Toxic Overload

Toxic Overload

A Doctor's Plan for Combating the Illnesses
Caused by Chemicals in Our Foods,
Our Homes, and Our Medicine Cabinets

Dr. Paula Baillie-Hamilton

Avery
a member of Penguin Group (USA) Inc.
New York

Published by the Penguin Group
www.penguin.com
Penguin Group (USA) Inc., 375 Hudson Street, New York, New York 10014, USA • Penguin Group
(Canada), 10 Alcorn Avenue, Toronto, Ontario M4V 3B2, Canada (a division of Pearson Penguin
Canada Inc.) • Penguin Books Ltd, 80 Strand, London WC2R 0RL, England • Penguin Ireland, 25
St Stephen's Green, Dublin 2, Ireland (a division of Penguin Books Ltd) • Penguin Group (Australia),
250 Camberwell Road, Camberwell, Victoria 3124, Australia (a division of Pearson Australia Group
Pty Ltd) • Penguin Books India Pvt Ltd, 11 Community Centre, Panchsheel Park, New Delhi–110
017, India • Penguin Group (NZ), Cnr Airborne and Rosedale Roads, Albany, Auckland 1310, New
Zealand (a division of Pearson New Zealand Ltd) • Penguin Books (South Africa) (Pty) Ltd,
24 Sturdee Avenue, Rosebank, Johannesburg 2196, South Africa
Penguin Books Ltd, Registered Offices: 80 Strand, London WC2R 0RL, England

Library of Congress Cataloging-in-Publication Data

Baillie-Hamilton, Paula.
Toxic overload : a doctor's plan for combating the illnesses caused by chemicals in our foods, our homes,
and our medicine cabinets / Paula Baillie-Hamilton.
p. cm.
Previously published in Great Britain as: Stop the 21st century killing you.
Includes bibliographical references and index.
ISBN 1-58333-225-1
1. Detoxification (Health)   2. Environmental toxicology.   3. Environmentally induced diseases.   I. Title.
RA784.5.B347   2005   2004062727
613—dc22

Printed in the United States of America
10 9 8 7 6 5 4 3 2 1

Book design by Lovedog Studio

This book is dedicated to
my dearly beloved husband, Mike,
and children, Angus, Bruce, Lucy, and Rory,

and to you and your children

Acknowledgments

It is a universally acknowledged fact that it is impossible to write a book without the support of others. So I would like to take this opportunity to thank all those who have played a pivotal role in the creation and production of this book.

The biggest thanks goes to Kristen Jennings, who with her excellent editorial advice transformed this book into what you have in your hands today. I am also very much indebted to Eric Levine for giving this book the full benefit of his remarkable PR creative skills.

Others I would like to thank are my sister Julia for her extremely constructive editorial advice and for all her excellent help and support every step of the way. My literary agent, Neeti Madan, my father, John Hickman, and mother, Pat Hickman, Professor Kim Jobst, my friend Elizabeth Kahn-Inglby, her daughter, Ella McHugh, Candida Rafferty, as well as all the oher people I have not mentioned who have played a role in supporting me personally or professionally in achieving my goals. Thank you all!

Contents

Introduction

Diseases once thought of as rare are now widespread. In 1900, less than 4 percent of the UK population died of heart disease and cancer combined. In 2002, this figure has increased to an unprecedented 65 percent.

TAKE A LOOK AT YOUR CLOTHES. We are now so used to buying fabrics in virtually any color under the sun that we take having this choice completely for granted. Yet our desire to wear beautifully colored clothes appears to have come at a terrible price, since it was the very creation of these bright, vibrant synthetic dyes which sparked the dawn of the modern-day chemical revolution.

Around 140 years ago, most dyes had to be created from naturally available products, so the range of colors was fairly limited. High prices excluded all but the richest people from buying cloth dyed with natural dyes. It was only when a chemist stumbled across a vibrant purple dye by using new and previously unknown methods of creating chemicals that scientists realized that a new era was within their control. This new "synthetic" dye not only possessed a new bright and attractive color, it was also cheaper, easier to produce, and more permanent than existing dyes, which tended to fade over time. In a nutshell, it possessed a range of more desirable, and therefore potentially profitable, characteristics than the existing natural dyes. Not surprisingly, not only did the chemist who discovered it soon make his fortune, but it prompted a modern-day gold rush driving large numbers of chemists to throw their efforts into using these revolutionary new methods in the hope that they, too, would discover new synthetic chemicals that could replace existing natural substances and earn them a fortune. Indeed man's endeavors in this field have been so vigorous that the chemical industry has snowballed into what is now the biggest industry in the world.

Indeed, not only are we now surrounded with hundreds of thousands of new synthetic chemicals, many of which are known to be highly toxic, but increased industrial use of toxic metals has also resulted in the unprecedented level of poisonous chemicals currently being released into our environment. With billions of kilograms of synthetic chemicals being produced annually in America alone, and with production doubling approximately every ten years, the situation appears to be escalating out of control.

We end up ingesting many of these chemicals, such as pesticides, preservatives, additives, pollutants, and contaminants, through our foods and food containers. We drink them in tap water, which contains chemicals leached from contaminated soils, environmental pollutants, and even chemicals added deliberately such as fluoride. We absorb them through our skin from cosmetics, toiletries, treated wood, sprayed plants, treated areas of public parks, golf courses, bath water, and swimming pools. We even inhale them in air contaminated with solvents, car fumes, industrial waste, and environmental pollutants.

The problem is that our bodies were never designed to protect themselves against this form of chemical onslaught. As a result, our systems usually fail to process and remove most of these chemicals once they have entered our bodies, so their levels start building up inside us. Consequently, every single human on the face of this earth is now permanently contaminated with these modern synthetic chemicals.

Unfortunately for our health, the greater the buildup of chemicals, the more pronounced their ability to disrupt the smooth running of our existing body systems. The consequences of this constant poisoning has, not surprisingly, been linked to the development and triggering of an ever-increasing number of diseases, such as asthma, autoimmune diseases, cancer, cardiovascular disease, diabetes, and thyroid diseases. Many leading scientists have hypothesized that these chemicals are now playing a significant role in perpetuating an epidemic of these and many other chronic illnesses.

Even over the last fifty years, the number of those with degenerative diseases has increased dramatically. People are developing diseases at younger ages, and the number of infants and children contracting chronic illnesses has never been higher. Furthermore, totally new illnesses, such as chronic fatigue syndrome, autism, and chemical sensitivities, have not only emerged but are already affecting a large percentage of the population. The pace of change has been so remarkable that the number of people affected by many of these diseases appears to be doubling every few decades.

As you can imagine, I am not the first scientist to question why these diseases have become so much more prevalent, as, to date, many billions of dollars have been spent in researching them. However, most of this research tends to focus on finding treatments rather than looking for causes. This has resulted in the development and marketing of an ever-increasing number of drugs designed to tweak the system and lessen aggravating symptoms, but, in most cases, not cure the disease itself.

So while the health of the pharmaceutical industry has never been better—according to MSNBC the combined profits for the ten drug companies in the Fortune 500 in 2002 was $35.9 billion, which was more than the profits for all the other 490 businesses combined—the health of the population has continued to plummet, and will continue to do so unless the actual causes of disease are tackled.

With every passing day, we seem to hear more and more reports linking our growing health problems to the increasing level of chemicals in our modern environment. Yet, despite these reports and the accompanying increasingly urgent warnings about these chemicals from scientists specializing in environmental medicine, the medical world appears to be deaf to these fears.

The reason for this widespread apathy originates in medical school, as few doctors are even taught about most modern-day chemicals. Perhaps fewer still are aware of how pervasive chemicals are, let alone understand the ways in which they could be poisoning us. As a result, during most medical consultations, the concept that chemical exposure may have contributed in some way to a patient's problem doesn't even enter the doctor's head. Doctors are trained to believe chemicals, i.e. drugs, are the answer, not the problem.

Consequently, not only do patients lose out on an opportunity to potentially reverse or minimize any chemically triggered problem, but some of the solutions offered by their doctors, pharmaceutical drugs, include highly toxic chemicals, such as pesticides and chemicals very similar to them, and may add to the overall problem.

This profound level of ignorance and general apathy on the part of the majority of the medical profession is what prompted me, a medical doctor and academic but also housewife and mother of four, to write this book. Through my study and research, I (along with a growing number of other highly qualified scientists) have been able to glimpse a world as yet unseen by the great majority of the medical profession.

An understanding of how toxic chemicals work and the knowledge of how to reverse their damaging effects is of extreme importance when dealing with all health issues. In my humble opinion, this knowledge could perhaps one day save your life.

Who This Book Will Help

Whether you currently have an illness that you wish to treat, are looking to optimize your existing health, or simply want to lower your chances of becoming ill in the future, this book is designed to help you achieve your health goals.

In Part I, after outlining the way certain chemicals contribute to disease and which lifestyles appear to be the most dangerous, I will set out my simple three-step plan that anyone can use as a foundation for creating his or her own individualized health programs.

➤ **Step One** outlines a supplement program essential to protecting your body from damage caused by toxic chemicals.

➤ **Step Two** explains how to rid your diet of toxins and concludes with a great seven-day plan to help shed your body's toxic load.

➤ **Step Three** identifies ways in which you can purge your home of toxins.

Part II of the book contains more specific information on a wide range of diseases, from Alzheimer's to autism and asthma. Not only will it tell you which chemicals are known to trigger or exacerbate certain diseases, it will also tell you how to deal with these diseases once you have developed them, as well as ways in which to protect yourself from these chronic illnesses in the first place.

Whatever your particular reason for being interested in your health, there are some truly amazing health benefits waiting to be discovered when you reduce your chemical toxicity. Not only will you greatly reduce existing disease symptoms, but you may also experience many healthy side effects of the program, such as weight loss, increased energy, less muscular and joint pain, a lower incidence of allergy symptoms, clearer thinking, improved digestion, a more positive outlook, and better skin and complexion. I now would like to wish you all good health and a very long life.

PART I

Beating Toxic Overload

CHAPTER 1

The Perils of a Polluted World

THE CREATION AND WIDESPREAD USE of man-made synthetic chemicals in the late twentieth century has resulted in every region of the planet being contaminated with a dangerous cocktail of known health-damaging toxins. The problem we now face is from the buildup of toxic effects these chemicals appear to be having on our health. With the average person being contaminated by an average of three hundred to five hundred industrial chemicals, the issue of how to deal with these unwanted intruders has become a problem for each and every one of us whether we like it or not

Ignoring the problem will not make it go away—all it will do is keep you ignorant of the many easy ways to effectively tackle health problems head on. This information could possibly save your life, and familiarizing yourself with the issues involved could be the best investment you will make in your health.

For most medical issues you can sit back and let someone else— probably your physician—take charge. However, if your physician or health care professional does not understand or know about the effect chemicals have on your health (and the odds are they will not), how can they possibly protect your health from the real dangers we all now face from chemicals? Unfortunately, defiant ignorance appears to be the position taken by most of the medical establishment on chemical toxicity. The growing problem that ever-increasing levels of toxic chemicals in the environment presents has become so complex, requiring learning a totally new set of treatment rules, that it has become easier to sweep the entire problem under the rug. Rather than waiting for the dinosaur of the medical establishment to catch up with the latest available information, the answer is to read about the many simple ways you can deal with this problem now. I think the best way to start is to know your enemy.

In this chapter, you will learn about the systems in your body that are responsible for flushing chemicals and toxins out of your body. It is the weakening of these systems by the onslaught of modern-day chemicals and pollutants that has led to the breakdown of the body's defenses against disease. This chapter will also introduce the major types of toxic chemicals in the environment and explain the short- and long-term effects of chemical exposure to your body. In chapters 2 through 4, you will learn the three easy steps to dramatically slash your exposure to the most toxic chemicals.

Our Detoxifying Systems

Our bodies have two goals when it comes to cleaning out its systems: (1) ridding the body of the waste products produced as by-products of its normal functions, and (2) detoxing and protecting our bodies from potentially harmful bacteria or toxic chemicals. Certain tissues play a vital role in removing unwanted substances, which if left unprocessed would quickly kill us. Most of the processing is done in our liver, which transforms toxins into harmless substances and mixes them into bile that is then released into the intestines for passage out of the body. Kidneys are also important detoxing organs, discarding waste in the urine. Our sinuses, skin, and lungs can also eliminate toxins through breath exhalation and sweating. But the liver is the body's most vital detoxifier, breaking down or transforming substances like ammonia, metabolic waste, drugs, alcohol, and chemicals that are present in the blood so that they can be excreted. There are two major detoxification pathways inside the liver cells: phase 1 and phase 2.

Phase 1 uses enzymes that reside on the membrane of the liver cells and convert toxic chemicals into less harmful substances through various chemical reactions such as oxidation, reduction, and hydrolysis. During any of these processes, free radicals are produced that, if excessive, can damage the liver cells. Antioxidants such as vitamins C and E and natural carotenoids reduce the damage caused by these free radicals. But, if antioxidants are lacking and toxin exposure is high, toxic chemicals become far more dangerous and some substances may be converted from relatively harmless compounds into potentially carcinogenic ones. Unfortunately, many substances, such as caffeine, alcohol, synthetic chemicals, saturated fats, pesticides, paint fumes, sulfonamides, exhaust fumes, and some drugs, also damage phase 1 detoxification pathways.

In the phase 2 detoxification pathway, called the "conjugation pathway," the liver cells add another substance (sulfur from certain amino acids or foods such as onions, eggs, and broccoli) to a toxic chemical or drug to render it less harmful. This pairing makes the toxin or drug water-soluble, allowing it to be excreted from the body via watery fluids such as bile or urine. Glutathione is a sulfur-containing protein that is the most powerful internal antioxidant and liver protector. Body levels of glutathione can be depleted by large amounts of toxins and/or drugs passing through the liver, as well as starvation or fasting. While phase 1 actions normally occur before phase 2 reactions, giving a lighter toxin load to the phase 2 system, this is not always the case. If the phase 1 and 2 detoxification pathways become overloaded, there will be an unhealthy buildup of toxins in the body.

Like all our other body systems, our detoxifying or waste disposal systems in our liver, kidneys, and body tissues will only work under the right circumstances, when our diets are high in unprocessed and nutritious foods. For hundreds of thousands of years our bodies used the relative abundance of nutrients and the naturally high fiber content of our diet to neutralize existing chemical threats. Today, we still need the same high levels of nutrients—such as vitamins, minerals, and essential fatty acids—and fiber to detoxify and remove chemicals. However, the world has moved on into unhealthy directions since these early days.

The Health Risk Posed by an Increasing Chemical Burden

Our modern, highly processed diets contain a fraction of the nutrients and fiber that they once did. This has resulted in the diverting of the few nutrients our bodies do get to systems that power our life support rather than those that flush out waste and chemical toxins. When you combine this with the explosive increase in the amount of heavy metals and synthetic chemicals in our food, homes, and beauty products, the result is that we are exposed to levels of chemicals far higher than our bodies were ever designed to withstand. This increase has effectively overloaded our natural coping mechanisms, which are now struggling to deal with their increased burden. The more saturated with chemicals these natural mechanisms become, the less able they are to protect us. The chemicals we can't process end up accumulating in our bodies and this growing toxic-chemical burden works to poison our tissues and exacerbate, as well as cause, disease.

Knowing this, it will probably come as no surprise that people with higher levels of toxic metals in their bodies are at a much greater risk of developing diseases such as cancer, cardiovascular disease, Alzheimer's, and diabetes, and that exposure to high levels of synthetic chemicals can make the situation even worse. Synthetic chemicals are not a part of nature, and our bodies' detoxification systems were not designed to deal with artificial chemicals—which include pesticides, drugs, chemicals containing chlorine and fluoride, plastics, and solvents. The synthetic properties of many chemicals make them impossible for our bodies to process or neutralize. The chemical-breakdown enzymes that make up part of our detoxification system simply fail to recognize, let alone work on, these new chemicals. Even if they are recognized as toxins by the body, because they are so durable, they continue to build up over time, unlike natural substances.

We already know that the average person's body burden of chemicals tends to increase throughout their lifetime. So as the level of chemicals poured into the environment rises to ever greater heights, the problem each one of us faces dealing with this new plague of chemical onslaught will continue to increase. It we don't start paying attention to the chemicals we are being increasingly exposed to and dealing with this issue proactively, our chances of remaining disease free for the rest of our lives will plummet.

There is an entire branch of medicine, known as environmental medicine, that deals with the health-damaging effects of toxic chemicals. Specialists in this field have carried out thousands of academic studies linking chemical exposure to a wide variety of diseases. Unfortunately, because very few health professionals learn about this subject during their training—I know that I certainly didn't when I was at medical school in the 1980s—this knowledge is only possessed by a relatively small number of highly specialized physicians who have spent years familiarizing themselves with the subject.

The barriers to knowledge are raised even higher by the dearth of readily available textbooks on the subject. This makes studying this field out of reach for most ordinary time-pressed physicians. I myself learned the hard way: To get to where I am today has taken many years of painstakingly gathering information from thousands of academic papers.

CHEMICAL POISONING

So how exactly do chemicals damage our health? Well, the harmful effects tend to be divided up into short-term and long-term damage. The most obvious and best-documented exposures are those where a person is effectively "poisoned" with a relatively large amount of chemicals. This triggers almost immediate and often violent symptoms. The symptoms experienced depend largely on the type of tissues damaged and the level and type of chemicals involved.

For instance, when the type of chemical commonly known as an organophosphate—found in nerve gas and in foods as a pesticide residue—comes into contact with muscle, it causes the structure of these tissues to actually dissolve. Indeed, these chemicals not only also kill muscle cells but also the nerves that control them, throwing the entire musculoskeletal system into disarray.

Their toxic actions fail to stop there as they also directly poison many glands, which produce hormones, thereby sending our natural body rhythm into total confusion. This extensive poisoning effect has led to organophosphates being one of the first chemicals developed for use as pesticides and chemical warfare weapons. Ironically, its efficiency as a killer is exactly what has made organophosphates one of the most common pesticide residues found in our foods.

Not surprisingly, the quicker and more dramatic poisoning episodes are relatively easy to recognize by the person affected and also by health professionals. Symptoms can range from mild flu-like illnesses to convulsions, unconsciousness, and death. Since these symptoms usually follow quickly after the poisoning incident, they are relatively well documented and on the whole hard to ignore. And, on a wider scale, these high-dose poisoning episodes account for a staggering 3 million cases of severe pesticide poisoning alone, including 220,000 fatalities worldwide every year. However, it is the more subtle form of long-term "low level" chemical poisoning that we will be concerned with in this book.

Long-Term Exposure

Lower dose chemical-induced health damage usually goes unnoticed by the affected person because disease development is often so slow and insidious. Warning signs of growing chemical damage are usually not recognized and are therefore ignored.

One of the primary mechanisms of chemical damage is called the "toxic chemical cocktail effect." The individual exposure levels of most chemicals are usually pretty low, meaning that their ability to individually damage the body is limited. However, the number of highly toxic chemicals our bodies are exposed to has dramatically increased in recent years, so it is not a question of our ability to deal with one or two chemicals, but with many thousands of them. Different chemicals tend to poison the same systems, though in a slightly different place, and the presence of one chemical could increase the toxicity of another chemical by ten or even one hundred or one thousandfold.

Since we already have hundreds of known chemicals in our bodies, the possibilities of health damage resulting from long-term exposure to the millions of different existing combinations of chemicals is immense. As such, the total effect of the toxic burden on the body is hard to estimate. While this makes research much more difficult, there are many ways in which the long-term health effects of chemicals can be discovered, such as by studying those exposed to high levels of certain types of chemicals—pesticides on pesticide workers or mercury on dental personnel. In this way, we can start to draw valuable connections between particular chemicals and particular illnesses.

Variables in the degree to which a person may experience toxic damage to their body include genetics, nutritional history, previous exposure to chemicals, and environment. Due to all of these circumstances, different people react in different ways to a given level of chemical exposure. Despite these uncertainties, the evidence that our long-term exposure to chemicals could be behind chronic illnesses is strong.

Not only is long-term exposure of toxic chemicals known to, and indeed intentionally used to, damage tissues, but their mere presence has been found to increase the amount of tissue-damaging free radicals in the body. In addition to this, the vast majority of chemicals also appear to be able to interfere with every single one of our major natural hormone systems. This hormonal damage stresses body systems, further increasing the chance of disease development.

A New Way of Thinking About Disease

Dr. Claudia Miller from the Department of Family Practice, University of Texas Health Science Center at San Antonio, believes that we are on the threshold of a new theory of disease, one that recognizes the impact of toxic chemicals. In a paper discussing chemical intolerance in *Annals of New York Academy of Sciences*, Miller wrote:

> In the late 1800s, physicians observed that certain illnesses spread from sick, feverish individuals to those contacting them, paving the way for the germ theory of disease. The germ theory served as a crude but elegant formulation that explained dozens of seemingly unrelated illnesses affecting literally every organ system.
>
> Today we are witnessing another medical anomaly—a unique pattern of illness involving chemically exposed people who subsequently report multisystem symptoms and new-onset chemical and food intolerances. These intolerances may be the hallmark for a new disease process, just as fever is a hallmark for infection.

So not only have chemicals now been linked with a large number of existing diseases, such as attention deficit disorder and cancer, but Miller and other prominent scientists believe this new disease process might be the key to explain the emergence of a totally new type of chemically related disorders, such as Gulf War syndrome, chronic fatigue syndrome, and chemical sensitivities.

The Chemicals Behind Our Health Problems

The chemicals that appear to be causing many current health problems can basically be divided into two main groups:

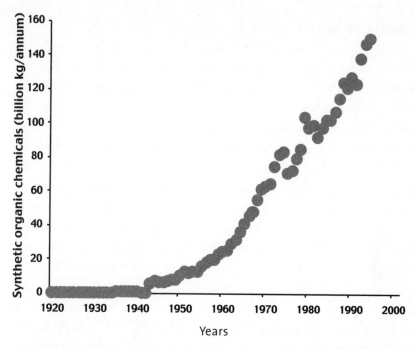

Figure 1. The Annual U.S. Production of Synthetic Chemicals, 1920–2000: Synthetic chemicals are extremely big business. Production in the United States alone in 1994 was worth a staggering $101 billion. The graph dramatically shows the phenomenal increase in production of these substances throughout the twentieth century.

➤ Toxic heavy metals and other toxic metals.
➤ Artificial or synthetic chemicals (halogens, organophosphates, carbamates, solvents, and plastics and plasticizers).

We are exposed to vast numbers of these toxins in everyday products. Although it would be impractical to go through all of them individually, I have picked out some of the most common chemicals and highlighted some of the places in which they can be found. The more you appreciate how widely these chemicals are used and their longevity, the more clearly you will understand why we are now so contaminated with them.

TOXIC METALS

Naturally occurring toxic metals, such as mercury, lead, cadmium, methyl mercury, and tributyltin (TBSPT), are used in a wide number of medical, dental, household, and industrial substances. There are other metals, such as aluminum, which, despite not being "strictly" heavy metals due to their atomic weight, possess a large number of toxic, health-damaging properties. Because these metals have been on the earth as long as we have, our bodies have had plenty of time to develop basic mechanisms of neutralizing and removing most of them. Our waste disposal systems are not only used in tackling toxic metals, but they have been designed to take on all forms of natural chemicals. However, the tendency of heavy metals to accumulate in the body over a lifetime of exposure makes them a cause of numerous health hazards.

Mercury has been proven to be an extremely health-damaging environmental substance, though it has often been used in industry and in the home. Just think of the phrase "as mad as a hatter," which became popular in the nineteenth century because many milliners exhibited strange behavior such as slurred speech and tremors. We now know that it was the mercury in the cloth used to make hats that caused these and other neurological symptoms. Today, as well as having been described as the second most toxic chemical in the world, mercury has been catagorized by Dr. Lars Friberg, MD, Ph.D., a former head of toxicology of the World Health Organization (WHO), in this way: "There is no safe level of mercury and no one has actually shown there is a safe level and I would say mercury is a very toxic substance."

Mercury's continued use in vaccine additives and dental amalgam on millions of unsuspecting people is utterly incomprehensible given mercury's extremely well-documented health risks. Unfortunately, most of us now have, on average, seven amalgam "silver" fillings. One filling contains approximately the same amount of mercury as a thermometer. We also know that mercury continually evaporates off all amalgam fillings at room temperature. This leakage increases dramatically with heat and trauma (e.g., by chewing hot foods). Indeed, using a phosphorescent screen you can actually see the mercury evaporating. And if

Everyday Sources of Toxic Heavy Metals

By avoiding toxic metals in these common sources, overall levels of lifetime mercury and aluminum contamination could be cut spectacularly. Common sources of heavy metals include:

Airborne metal particles near mines, smelters, and metal processing or heavy engineering works (all metals)

Carbonated beverages in aluminum cans (aluminum)

Cooking utensils (aluminum)

Dental amalgam (mercury, tin, silver, copper)

Electroplating (most metals)

Food additives (aluminum)

Food contaminants (mercury, lead, TBT, arsenic, cadmium in seafood and shellfish)

Glass (lead, antimony)

Lead building materials, cable covering, and roofing

Lead plumbing (lead pipes and copper pipes joined by lead solder)

Nickel plating for soldering, in alloys, photoelectric cells, and storage batteries (cadmium is also found in batteries)

Paint additive (lead, TBT, cadmium, antimony)

Products containing lead (lead crystal, pottery with lead ceramic glazes, stained glass windows joined with strips of lead, old painted toys)

Tap water (aluminum is used as a cleaning agent in water processing plants)

Vaccine additives (mercury, aluminum)

you can see it, mercury levels in the air will already be at least 1,000 times higher than the Environmental Protection Agency's (EPA) "safe level in air" guidelines. (To see evidence of this "smoking teeth" effect, go to the International Academy of Oral Medicine and Toxicology's Web site at www.iaomt.com.)

In 1991 the WHO stated that for most people, daily exposure to mercury is through their dental fillings—which can expose people to more than eight times the amount of mercury as is found in all other major sources such as seafoods. Indeed the existing research is so overwhelming that it has led to the banning of mercury in dental amalgam

Health Problems Associated with Mercury Poisoning

Excessive flow of saliva

Inflammation of mouth and gums

Irritability

Jerky gait

Kidney damage

Learning disabilities

Loosening of teeth

Muscle tremors

Nervousness

Personality changes

Pins and needles

Spasms of extremities

Swelling of salivary glands

in many countries. However, despite all this, somewhat incredibly, thousands of American dentists will continue to pile yet more tons of mercury into people's mouths.

The problem of deliberate contamination with these heavy metals does not stop there: Mercury and aluminum are regularly injected into people's bodies in the form of vaccine adjuvants. The main purpose of adjuvants is to make vaccines cheaper as they reduce the amount of headline antigen (such as tetanus) that needs to be used for the vaccine to be effective: the adjuvant artificially revs up the immune system, falsely sending it into overdrive to fight off disease or infection. Toxic metals have been used as adjuvants for decades because, in addition to being comparatively cheap, they are extremely good at damaging the immune system. In addition to the immediate damage caused by injecting extremely high levels of toxic metals, this excessive immune system

Health Problems Associated with Aluminum Poisoning

Abnormal EEG

Alzheimer's disease

Anemia

Blood clots

Bone disorders, including fractures

Coarse tremors

Heart attack

Learning disabilities

Mental status changes

Speech disturbances

Stroke

disturbance continues long after the vaccine has been given. It can actually last as long as the toxic metals remain in our bodies, which can be for decades because they can get locked into our tissues— particularly our brains and bones.

Unfortunately, the childhood vaccination program in the United States has meant that children who received all of the recommended vaccinations between 1989 and 1999 would have absorbed the "safe" amount of mercury recommended for their entire lifetime by the time they were six months old. This "mistake" was so serious that it even prompted an adviser to the National Immunization Program, Dr. Neal Halsey of Johns Hopkins University, at a hearing in Cambridge three years ago, to admit, "I feel badly that I didn't pick it up." While mercury has now been removed from all routine childhood vaccines, at the time of this writing it is still present in many nonroutinely adminis-

Health Problems Associated with Lead Poisoning

Anorexia

Antisocial behavior

Convulsions

Loss of IQ in children or thinking abilities in adults

Mental confusion

Nausea

Paralysis

Severe abdominal pain and anemia

Visual disturbances

Vomiting

tered childhood vaccines and adult vaccines, such as the flu and meningitis vaccines.

Carbonated drinks stored in aluminum cans are a significant source of aluminum contamination. Because aluminum tends to dissolve in acidic and salty fluids, the level of aluminum contamination will be related to the amounts of these substances in the drink.

HALOGENS AND THEIR COMPOUNDS

Chlorine, fluorine, and bromine are all halogens, substances we are all regularly exposed to either in a simple compound or as part of a more complex, artificially manufactured, synthetic chemical such as organochlorine, organobromine, and other organohalogens.

Like toxic metals, these naturally occurring chemicals appear to play a significant role in either triggering or exacerbating many chronic diseases. Not only are halogens individually toxic, many chemicals in which these substances are used are considered a serious health hazard. For evidence of this, you only have to look at what they have been used for. For instance, chlorine is notorious for its use as a potent war gas and as a pesticide. It has also been used as an additive to virtually every major water supply in the United States as a water disinfectant. The extremely toxic gas fluorine began to be manufactured seriously in World War II as it was essential for the nuclear bomb project and nuclear energy applications, and its presence is also extremely common in pesticides. Bromine is widely used in pesticides due to its natural toxicity. Like chlorine and fluoride, many of the compounds that contain these halogens have been either banned or severely restricted due to the extreme health danger they pose to humans.

When halogens such as chlorine are attached to more complicated synthetic compounds, they are converted into organochlorine, organobromine, and other organohalogens. This group is particularly important due to the total inability of our bodies to "see" and therefore rid itself of them. Our inability to process these halogens, combined with their innate ability to damage living tissues, is not only the reason they started to be used so extensively as pesticides in the first place, but is

Health Problems Associated with Halogens

The toxicities from fluorine and its compounds, such as the organofluorines, are extremely numerous, with the main health problems including the following:

Anemia

Bone damage

Brain damage, particularly in children

Cancer

Heart arrhythmias

Hormonal damage

Hyperactivity in children

Immune-system damage such as lowered immunity

Increased cholesterol

Kidney damage

Reduced energy

Reduced IQ

Thin hair and skin

Weight problems (both weight loss and obesity)

also related to what makes these synthetic organohalogens such a major health problem now.

Most developed countries have banned many types of organochlorine pesticides now, but owing to their previous extensive use and their long-lasting effects, their production is thought to have resulted in the permanent pollution of the entire planet. They can still enter our bodily

Everyday Sources of Halogens

Disinfectants and cleaning solutions

Dyes

Gasoline

Medicines (about 85 percent of all pharmaceuticals contain or are manufactured with chlorine)

Pesticide residue in foods

Photograph developing solutions

Toothpaste

Water purification processes

Health Problems Associated with Synthetic Halogen Compounds

Behavioral problems

Brain disorders

Cancer

Depression

Diabetes

High cholesterol

Immune system disorders

Infertility

Thyroid disease

Widespread toxicity to the body's hormonal systems

Sources of Synthetic Halogen Compounds

Adhesives

Anti-malaria spray

Carbonless duplicating paper

Carpets (pesticides from wool carpets) and vinyl flooring

Combusted leaded petroleum products

Common herbicides

DDT (a now-banned pesticide that is still widely present as an environmental pollutant)

Dioxin (an industrial waste by-product and one of the most toxic chemicals ever produced)

Electrical conductors

Inks

Insecticides and fungicides

Medicines

Nit shampoo and treatments for head and crab lice

Paints and dyes (oil- and water-based)

PBB (used as a fire retardant in fabrics, clothes, curtains, furniture coverings, and wood)

PCB (previously used as an insulating fluid in electrical equipment)

Pesticides

Surface coatings

Wood preservatives and treatment for termite protection

systems as environmental pollutants, especially through the consumption of contaminated animal fats in fish and fish oil. Furthermore, these pesticides continue to be produced and used in developing countries, largely because of their relatively low cost, even though many of their dangers are well known.

Although the estimated health risk from our exposure to these halogen-containing compounds is varied, their universal presence, their often extreme stability combined with our relative inability to break down and excrete many of them from our bodies has led me to give these substances a high risk rating. There are many serious, and even life-threatening, immediate health risks due to high-level exposure to these compounds, such as inflammation of the lungs, seizure, and unconsciousness. However, most people suffer from long-term, low-level exposure.

ORGANOPHOSPHATES

Organophosphates are synthetically manufactured chemicals that were developed as a nerve gas and used in the Second World War. Since

Health Problems Associated with Organophosphates

Anxiety

Confusion

Depression

Emotional lability

Irritability

Lethargy

Loss of concentration

(continued)

Health Problems Associated with Organophosphates

Memory loss

Paralysis

Problems identifying words, colors, or numbers, and an inability to speak fluently

Severe fatigue

Common Sources of Organophosphates

Animal growth promoters

Cattle treatments

Flame retardants

Flea treatments for pets (shampoos, sprays, powders, flea collars)

Gasoline additives

Household and garden pesticides such as fly spray

Medicines, particularly treatment for lice, crabs, and nits, and Alzheimer's disease

Pesticides for crops, particularly soft fruit, vegetables, and grain products

Rubber additives

Sheep dips

Stabilizers in lubricating and hydraulic oils

Synthetic additives

Wood infestation treatments

then, they have been used very extensively in many different areas of manufacturing, food production, and even medicine. They are now some of the most common pesticides detected in our foods.

The estimated health risk of organophosphates is high. Although the toxicity of organophosphates varies, they are some of the most powerful pesticides in current usage and damage a variety of different body systems. Serious health risks can result due to high-level, short-term exposure, but low-level, short-term exposure is more common. Long-term exposure also exacerbates diseases of the heart such as arrhythmias as well as high cholesterol, cancer, allergies, and diseases of hormonal systems, particularly the thyroid gland, and the immune system.

CARBAMATES

The actions of synthetically manufactured carbamates are thought to be similar to those of organophosphates, but are generally considered

Common Sources of Carbamates

Animal growth promoters

Anti-microbials

Cigarettes and cigars

Flea treatments for pets (all kinds)

Forestry and wood infestation treatments

Fungicides

Herbicides

Insecticides

Metal chelating agents

Mothballs

Synthetic rubber

to be less toxic. Because of this similarity, they produce many of the same symptoms as organophosphates in the body. Some effects last for a shorter period than those of organophosphates, but other toxic actions can last for much longer periods and result in permanent damage. They are known particularly to lower our energy levels as they target our metabolism.

Carbamates have been used as growth promoters in a battery of farm situations because of their ability to slow down the overall metabolic rate. They are used in medicine for their anti–thyroid hormone actions because they slow thyroid functions. As they are added to foods after harvesting, in the form of fungicides, they tend to be present in relatively large quantities in a wide range of foods including potatoes, citrus fruits, peanuts, and tomatoes. Their health risk to the average person on a nonorganic diet is moderate to high.

SOLVENTS

These synthetically manufactured chemicals are widely used in a range of products, including many volatile organic compounds, or VOCs. Solvents are used extensively throughout industry to dissolve or dilute oils and fats and as a petroleum additive, as well as being used in numerous home products such as toiletries, food packaging, and floor waxes.

The estimated health risk of solvents is moderate, but they are found in abundance in the environment. They appear to play a role in many chronic illnesses, but they are particularly harmful to the brain due to their extreme solubility in fats. This can result in memory loss, Alzheimer's, and other types of brain disorders.

PLASTICS AND PLASTICIZERS

Common plastic additives include phthalates, a substance that makes plastics flexible, and bisphenol, which is used to line food packaging. Since plastics are so widely used, phthalates and bisphenols are now said to be the most abundant industrial contaminants in the environment. At room temperature, phthalates evaporate from products that contain them, producing that characteristic "new plastic" smell.

Common Sources of Solvents

Aftershaves

Detergents

Dry-cleaning fluids

Floor wax

Household pesticides

Latex

Metal foils used in food packaging (e.g., yogurt lids)

Perfumes

Polystyrene cups, plates, and packaging

Resin

Skin-care products such as "natural" or "botanical" creams and lotions

Synthetic rubber

Toiletries

The estimated health risk posed by these plastic additives is moderate. Although these can mostly be metabolized in the body, their extensive presence ensures that they are a constant source of metabolic and hormonal disruption in our bodies. PVC (vinyl) is thought to be the worst kind of plastic. Not only is it made with chlorine, but it also releases dioxins (toxic hydrocarbons) throughout its lifetime. Dioxins have been linked to cancer (such as breast, prostate, and immune system), hormonal imbalances (thyroid gland, infertility), high blood pressure, heart disease, autoimmune diseases, weight problems, and chronic fatigue.

Common Sources of Plastics and Plasticizers

Adhesives and glues

Carpet backing

Cleaning compounds derived from petroleum

Cosmetics, perfumes, shampoo, hair products, and nail polish

Detergents

Fatty foods such as eggs, dairy, and breast milk

Fish

Food wrapping and containers

Household pesticides and insect repellants

Industrial cleaning agents

Inks

Lining of cardboard, metal, and aluminum food containers

Lubricants and corrosion inhibitors

Paints (oil- and water-based)

Plastic bottles

Synthetic rubber and plastic products

Synthetic leather

Tubing

Vinyl (PVC) and all types of plastics

Water pipes

Waterproof clothing

How Great Is Your Exposure to Health-Damaging Chemicals?

Below is a checklist of the most hazardous lifestyle factors, in descending order of toxicity, that can cause an accumulation of toxic chemicals in your body. Go down the list, marking off any items that apply to you. The more that apply to you, the greater your exposure to disease-causing chemicals.

___ The presence of mercury amalgam or "silver" dental fillings.

___ Living in an old house with lead-based paints and with water pipes made of lead (or with copper pipes and lead solder).

___ Being vaccinated with vaccines containing mercury or aluminum. (The greater the number of vaccines given, the higher the level of potential contamination.)

___ Previous dental work which involved removing or inserting mercury amalgam fillings.

___ An existing or previous job or pastime working with synthetic chemicals (such as hairdressing, farming), solvents (such as painting and decorating or dry cleaning), or toxic metals (such as welding), and halogens (such as bromine from developing photographs).

___ Previous and current usage of concentrated forms of chemical pesticides and herbicides around your house and garden (fly spray, weed killer, flea powder).

___ Exposure to chemicals in medicines (nit shampoo, certain drugs, skin whiteners, etc.).

___ Smoking (tobacco contains a wide number of cancer-causing chemicals which include toxic metals).

___ Using nonenvironmentally friendly cosmetics, such as deodorants (which contain aluminum), toiletries, such as hairsprays, perfumes, nail varnish, etc. (which contain solvents and plastics).

___ Using fluoridated toothpaste.

____ Using nonenvironmentally friendly household cleaners.

____ Living in a major city (due to air pollution).

____ Eating the skins or outside leaves of conventionally grown fruits and vegetables (nonorganic, particularly strawberries, apples, pears, carrots, lettuce).

____ Regularly drinking one or more soft drinks from aluminum cans a day.

____ A diet that consists mostly of processed foods (due to the use of artificial preservatives, colorings, flavorings, and additives).

____ The regular intake of sugar-free or low-sugar foods and drinks, which use artificial sweeteners (such as aspartame and saccharine).

____ Eating a large amount of seafood (as seafoods tend to be contaminated both with toxic metals and organochlorines).

____ Living near fields that are regularly sprayed with pesticides.

____ Drinking and bathing in unfiltered tap water (due to the deliberately added aluminum and chlorine disinfectant, fluorine, and the general water contaminants).

Where to Go From Here

The good news is that by making simple lifestyle changes, it is possible to significantly lower the level of toxic chemicals in your body. Throughout the rest of Part I, I will guide you through three simple steps for ridding your food, home, and body of dangerous toxins that contribute to disease. First, I will outline a nutritional supplement program that will boost your body's natural ability to kick out toxins and act as an internal sponge, soaking up more persistent toxins so that they can then be expelled from the body. Second, I will explain the benefits of organic foods and teach you food preparation methods that will greatly reduce the amount of chemicals you consume through your diet. I will also give you my Seven-Day Desludge Diet, which provides a complete menu plan that will help cleanse your system and put you on the track to protecting yourself from chemical-induced ill-

The Three Steps to a Chemical-Free Life

Step 1. The Detoxifying Supplement Program
Step 2. Seven-Day Desludge Diet
Step 3. Detoxing Your Home

nesses. Third, I will teach you valuable tips for detoxifying your home of common household chemicals and toxins.

Through these three steps, you will reduce your exposure to the most concentrated sources of toxins, lower your existing body burden of dangerous health-damaging chemicals, and minimize your future exposure.

Some of these tips may take some time for you to implement. But the key is to do what you can when you can. The fact of the matter is that these chemicals are simply not going to go away, so we need to adapt to this polluted world if we are to survive.

The good news is that we can all enjoy better health just by knowing the new rules—if you understand what the problem is then you hold the key to the solution. A little effort focused in the right places will greatly assist you in achieving a healthier and more vibrant body and lifestyle, despite the proliferation of synthetic chemicals and other hazards. Follow these tips at your own pace—even if you take up just one of these suggestions, it will make a difference.

CHAPTER 2

Step 1.
Supplementation

WHILE CHEMICAL AVOIDANCE WILL PLAY a critical role in ridding your body of disease-causing toxins, starting a long-term daily supplement program is vital for relieving your body of its existing burden of chemicals and protecting you from future chemical exposure. Many studies show that the most effective way of detoxing is by fortifying and powering our own natural detoxification systems, which consist of a vast array of tissues and enzymes that work round the clock to neutralize and rid our bodies of toxic substances (see chapter 1). Because our detox systems rely on the presence of a wide range of nutrients to be fully functional, we need to ensure that our levels of all the most important vitamins and minerals are optimized at all times.

The prominence of nutritional supplements in the detox program is due to the fact that the mere presence of artificial chemicals appears to have increased the need for nutrients to the point that we now need more vitamins and minerals than we can realistically get from our diet. Consequently, most people are deficient in at least one or more essential nutrients. Adding to the problem, the foods in our diets provide fewer nutrients than they used to. Many factors in modern food growth, consumption, and processing have contributed to this change, including:

➤ "Conventional" farming methods that tend to produce nutrient-deficient foods, as opposed to traditional organic farming methods.

➤ Increased food storage and transportation time, which increases nutrient depletion.

➤ Food processing and refinement that destroys nutrients.

➤ An increase in the amount of processed foods consumed by the average American.

Many scientists now believe that everyone needs to have a higher intake of nutrients than their diet accounts for in order to improve body functioning, deal with the body's chemical load, and to prevent and treat illnesses. The Toxic Overload program involves taking a good multivitamin and mineral supplement, as well as magnesium, vitamin C, essential fatty oils, MSM-sulphur, probiotics, and fiber.

While the daily detox supplement program provided in this chapter has been designed to suit the needs of the majority of people, the variability in lifestyle, diet, and genetic inheritance means that not everyone's needs are the same. As a result, some people may need higher levels of certain nutrients than others. You can find out more about the particular nutritional demands that different diseases pose at the end

Why We Now Need More Nutrients Than Ever Before

➤ To protect our tissues from chemical-induced free radicals.

➤ To power our bodies' detoxification systems, allowing them to process, neutralize, and eliminate toxic chemicals.

➤ To repair and prevent direct damage from synthetic chemicals to body tissues.

➤ To replenish the increased loss of nutrients from our bodies' stores triggered by toxic chemicals.

of the appropriate chapters in Part II, but it is also possible to be tested and to have a program designed for your specific needs. To find a physician who can test your nutritional status, visit the Web site of the American Academy of Environmental Medicine at www.aaem.com.

Getting the Most from Your Multivitamin

The levels of various vitamins and minerals needed can vary dramatically among individuals according to need, whether or not they are taking medication, their exposure to chemicals, and the presence of disease. In addition, many people use nutrients over a short term for therapeutic purposes and take higher levels than they might take over the long term. Because of this, nutrient levels can only ever be approximate.

However, a good multivitamin and mineral supplement can provide appropriate levels of virtually all of the nutrients vital to health and essential for detoxing the body. With our need for nutrients continually rising as a result of our ever-increasing chemical burden, nutrient-poor foods, frantic lifestyles, and perpetual food-restricting diets, taking a multivitamin is essential to health and is the bedrock of any supplement program. The sidebar "Levels of Vitamins and Minerals Desired in a Multivitamin" (page 41) outlines the vitamins and minerals you should look for when buying a multivitamin and in what quantities. To fully detox and protect yourself from chemical damage, it may be necessary for you to take additional supplements of some vitamins, such as vitamin C. The "Daily Supplement Program" sidebar (page 50) details precisely how much of each supplement, including your multivitamin, you should take daily.

It is also of vital importance to get the *right* multivitamin and mineral supplement, since the dosages of many are lower than many scientists now believe necessary, as they were calculated without taking into consideration the increased need due to the presence of chemicals. (See Resources for reputable supplement companies.) Below is some information on some of the most important chemical detoxifiers, all of which will be found in a good multivitamin.

Vitamin A and Other Antioxidants

Carotenes are converted in the body to vitamin A, which is essential for good eyesight and night vision, bone formation and normal body growth, especially of the skin and teeth, and health during pregnancy and lactation. As an antioxidant, vitamin A helps soak up damaging free radicals that are released when chemicals come into contact with body tissues. It also detoxifies the body; protects against cancer, heart disease, and other diseases; and enhances immune system function. Food sources include meat; milk and milk products; cereal products; eggs; fish; dark green, dark yellow, and orange vegetables; carrots; sweet potatoes; peaches; oranges; and apples.

Commonly found chemicals, such as PCBs, solvents, insecticides, and drugs, can dramatically drain body stores of vitamin A and other antioxidants by increasing its usage and excretion. Our exposure to toxins has dramatically increased our demand for these tissue-protecting antioxidants. This can lead to an increased instance of many diseases. For example, 20 percent of people with chemical sensitivities tend to have deficient blood levels of vitamin A. Also, people who are deficient in antioxidants are at a higher risk of developing chronic diseases such as asthma, cancer, cardiovascular disease, and diabetes. Many medical conditions show benefit from vitamin A supplementation, including allergies; skin, gum, and mouth complaints; asthma; visual problems; and an increased vulnerability to infections.

Plant-based carotenes are nontoxic, even when consumed in large amounts over long periods of time, except that harmless, temporary yellowing of skin occurs. However, heavy smokers, due to their extremely low levels of vitamin C, should not take very high levels of beta-carotene by itself, as the resulting imbalance in those who do not take enough vitamin C could increase free radicals. Vitamin A found in animal-derived foods is toxic only in prolonged excessive intake and can cause birth defects. If trying to conceive, do not exceed 3,000 mcg retinol (10,000 IUs) or 3,000–30,000 mcg beta-carotene per day.

A good multivitamin and mineral will include the most important antioxidants: vitamins A, C, and E, coenzyme Q10, and the minerals selenium and zinc. Other antioxidants include the omega-3 oils and the "detoxing" amino acid known as glutathione (see pages 45–46).

B Vitamins

Our bodies need large amounts of the B group of vitamins—B_1, B_6, and B_{12} in particular—in order to process toxic chemicals. These nutrients also play an important role in powering our metabolism and preventing a wide range of diseases and conditions (such as high cholesterol) from developing. Most people who are exposed to a large amount of chemicals tend to be grossly deficient in these nutrients.

Vitamin B_1 (thiamin) contributes to the normal functioning of all body cells, especially nerves. It aids the metabolism of carbohydrates, protein, and fats for energy, and is a vital detoxer. Up to 30 percent of people sensitive to chemicals are deficient in vitamin B_1. Vitamin B_1 appears to be particularly useful in the treatment of muscle disorders, indigestion, mental illness, diabetes, depression, fatigue, excessive chemical toxicity, and failure to detoxify chemicals. Food sources include potatoes, wheat germ, nutritional yeast, cooked beans and peas, collard greens, raisins, oranges, nuts, whole grains, milk, and milk products.

Vitamin B_6 aids in formation and maintenance of the nervous system and immune system, the regulation of mental processes and mood, and is vital in chemical detoxification. Approximately 60 percent of people with chemical sensitivities are deficient in vitamin B_6. Unfortunately, in addition to being one of the most important key nutrients with respect to our entire metabolism and detoxification system, it appears to be one of the most vulnerable to deficiency due to increased usage and problems with absorption. Food sources include cooked dried beans and peas, nutritional yeast, beef liver, wheat germ, nuts, bananas, avocados, leafy greens, cabbage, cauliflower, potatoes, whole grains, dried fruit, fish, and venison. Supplementation through a multivitamin is essential in most cases to ensure sufficient levels are received. Vitamin B_6 is toxic to the nervous system when taken in supplements in doses above 1,000 milligrams.

Levels of Vitamins and Minerals Desired in a Multivitamin

Essential Supplements	Total Daily Amount
Vitamin A* (retinol or beta-carotene)	5,000–10,000 IU
Vitamin C	60 mg
Vitamin D	400–800 IU
Vitamin E**	40–400 IU
Thiamin	3–25 mg
Riboflavin	1.8–25 mg
Niacin	25–50 mg
Vitamin B_6	5–25 mg
Folic acid	400–1,000 mcg
Vitamin B_{12}	2–50 mcg
Biotin	50–300 mcg
Pantothenic acid	25–50 mg
Calcium	500–1,000 mg
Phosphorus	350—1,000 mg
Iodine	150 mcg
Magnesium	300–500 mg
Zinc	15–30 mg
Selenium	50–100 mcg
Iron***	15–18 mg

IU = international units; mcg = micrograms; mg = milligrams; 1,000mcg = 1mg

*If pregnant or trying to conceive, do not exceed 10,000 IU of preformed vitamin A each day.

**If you have high blood pressure or are taking blood thinners (anticoagulant medication) start with 100 IU and consult your doctor.

*** Adult men and postmenopausal women may not need supplemental iron, unless they have previous or existing raised exposure to lead contamination.

Vitamin C

Vitamin C (ascorbic acid) is one of the best-known antioxidant and free-radical scavengers around. This water-soluble vitamin plays a vital role in protecting our bodies from the continual damage chemicals inflict on it. The importance of this critical nutrient is readily demonstrated in the hundreds of academic papers that consistently reveal that the lower the intake of vitamin C, the greater the chance of developing numerous chronic illnesses.

Research also reveals that taking vitamin C can lower the severity of disease and reduce the risk of developing many illnesses in the first place. Vitamin C supplementation can also help tackle many existing immune system and health problems by speeding up wound and burn healing, reducing recovery times after surgery, lowering chemical sensitivities, increasing energy levels, relieving symptoms and muscle pain in chronic fatigue syndrome, reducing the risk of developing cancer, helping to prevent lead poisoning, protecting against heart disease, enhancing mobility and improving arthritis and rheumatic tissue disorders, lowering blood cholesterol, and reducing blood clotting.

Vitamin C is naturally found in peppers, citrus fruits, tomatoes, melons, broccoli, and green leafy vegetables such as spinach, and turnip and mustard greens. However, don't rely on eating an orange a day to give you enough of this nutrient as one study showed that "fresh" oranges bought from some vendors contained no vitamin C at all due to to the excessive amount of time they had been stored. So to ensure you get all the vitamin C you need, it's best to supplement your diet. Because multivitamins do not usually contain the level of vitamin C we need (it would make them too bulky), we need to take an additional vitamin C supplement to get a total of 500 mg to 2000 mg each day. Vitamin C only stays in the body for eight to twelve hours, so to ensure twenty-four hour protection it's best to divide your daily dose of vitamin C, taking half in the morning and the other half in the evening.

Magnesium

Magnesium appears to be one of the most important minerals required for chemical detoxification, as it protects the body's tissues, particularly the brain, from the toxic effects of heavy and other toxic metals such as mercury and aluminum. It is probable that low levels of total body magnesium contribute to the toxic metal deposition in the brain that precedes Parkinson's, multiple sclerosis, Alzheimer's disease, and learning disorders. Magnesium also plays a major role in aiding the smooth functioning of hormones such as insulin, thyroid, estrogen, testosterone, and catecholamines, and it controls the proper absorption and retention of calcium in the body. Magnesium is also known as the "relaxing" mineral for its ability to relax muscle tissue and prevent it from going into spasm, thereby easing airway constriction in asthma and dilating blood vessels to lower blood pressure. Indeed, it is a critical element in more than 325 biochemical reactions in the human body.

Unfortunately, due to food processing and modern agriculture practices, the amount of magnesium in the standard diet is low, and a very large percentage of people have suboptimal or deficient levels of magnesium. Magnesium deficiency is so common and causes so many health problems that there is an entire medical journal dedicated to this vital mineral.

Common food sources of magnesium include wheat germ, all nuts and seeds, tofu, broccoli, spinach, Swiss chard, soybeans, tomato paste, all beans, brewer's yeast, sweet potatoes, squash, avocados, bananas, dark green leafy vegetables, yogurt, and milk. Supplementation is often highly effective in treating or allieviating many problems, such as high blood pressure, cholesterol, depression, anxiety attacks, heart failure, heart attacks, kidney stones, childhood behavioral disorders, obesity, tooth decay, lead poisoning, and failure to detoxify chemicals.

Omega-3 Oils

While many people are used to taking vitamin and mineral supplements, comparatively few take essential oils, yet these nutrients are vital to good health. Omega-3 and omega-6 oils are found in every cell of our bodies and they play an important part in normal functioning of all body

Possible Reaction to Detoxing

If your body is particularly run down or nutrient deficient, you might feel temporarily worse for a few weeks after you begin your supplement program before you begin to feel better. Symptoms may include getting a cold or other infection, feeling very tired, or experiencing a flare-up of an existing complaint. This is because for the first time in years, the body will actually have sufficient resources to start dealing with the massive buildup of stored chemicals. The temporary ill effects are thought to be caused by the increased mobilization of chemicals that are in the process of breaking down.

Don't be disheartened if this happens to you. On the contrary, you should realize that it is happening because the supplements are having the desired effect. Keep going and this phase will soon wear off. You will soon be rewarded with a higher level of health.

tissues. These essential oils can also help prevent atherosclerosis; reduce incidence of heart disease, depression, and stroke; and bring relief from the symptoms associated with ulcerative colitis, menstrual pain, and joint pain. They also help detoxify chemicals in the body, increase energy levels, reduce inflammation, and keep skin supple. People deficient in these health-giving oils are not only less able to detoxify chemicals, but are also much more prone to developing a wide number of different diseases.

Food sources of omega-3 fatty acids include nuts, seeds, vegetables, beans, and fruits; vegetable oils such as canola, flaxseed, soybean, walnut, and wheat germ; and salmon, halibut, sardines, albacore, trout, and herring. Other foods that contain omega-3 fatty acids include shrimp, clams, chunk light tuna, catfish, cod, and spinach. But, because many people have a low intake of foods that contain high levels of these nutrients, a daily supplement is advisable. Most omega-3 supplements contain a small amount of omega-6 oils as well, so it is not necessary to take an extra omega-6 supplement.

Omega-3 supplements made from vegetable oils such as flax and hemp tend to be relatively free from chemicals and make a good choice for supplementation over the relatively polluted fish oils. However, a small group of people are unable to convert vegetable oils into oils that their body can use, so fish oils would be the oils of choice for them. Only testing can tell you if you are able to convert these oils; however, if you are taking all the other supplements and seeing improvements in your energy, health, and skin after a few weeks on the vegetable-based oils, the chances are that you have no problem in processing them. If you don't want to risk it and want to reduce the amount of oil you need to take a day, you can buy brands such as Dr. Sear's OmegaRx Ultra-Refined fish oil, or my personal favorite brand, Nordic Naturals, which have had the chemicals removed by a distillation process. The latter can be found in most good health food stores. When taking fish oils, follow dosage recommendations found on the package. There is a wide variability in potency between brands, so I cannot offer a general guideline here.

When purchasing an omega-3 fatty acid supplement, remember that these oils are highly sensitive to damage from heat, light, and oxygen. Choose a certified organic or chemical-free product that has been refrigerated and is packaged in a dark brown or green glass jar, and be sure to store the product in your refrigerator or freezer.

Amino Acids and MSM-sulphur

One of the problems with chemical pollutants is that they damage the way our bodies break down, absorb, use, and manufacture amino acids. In fact, many people who get adequate amounts of amino acids in their diet remain deficient due to the antinutrient effects of chemicals. Certain amino acids are crucial to our ability to detoxify ourselves of chemical pollutants, particularly the harder to shift organochlorines. The amino acids that should be taken as supplements include methionine, cysteine, taurine, and glutathione.

Glutathione is a powerful antioxidant that helps detox the liver of poisonous chemicals, especially alcohol and mercury. It also protects against damage caused by exposure to pesticides, plastics, smoke, nitrates, and drugs. Glutathione also helps to prevent aging, AIDS, cancer, cataracts, infertility, Parkinson's disease, rheumatoid arthritis, schizophrenia, and heavy-metal poisoning (arsenic, lead, mercury), and helps prevent ulcers caused by medications such as NSAIDS (nonsteroidal anti-inflammatory drugs). Food sources include fresh fruits and vegetables, especially asparagus and avocados, and fresh meats.

Amino acids can be found in many of the foods in the Seven-Day Desludge Diet, but to ensure that you are receiving optimal levels you might add a supplement, but do not take very high doses (no more than 7 g per day). Patients with cystinuria, a genetic abnormality which causes the defective absorption of the amino acid cystine, and can lead to the development of kidney and bladder stones, should not take it. Persons with liver or kidney diseases should seek their doctor's approval before taking amino acid supplements.

For those who want to minimize their intake of supplements, MSM-sulfur (MSM stands for methylsulfonylmethane) could prove an alternative to taking amino acids. This is because MSM, a natural form of sulfur, combined with a good supply of vitamins and minerals, can boost the body's natural ability to create these sulfur-containing amino acids.

I have added this fabulous antioxidant to the program because it appears to play an essential role in cleaning up and safely removing some of the most persistent heavy metals, such as mercury, from the body. It also lowers allergies to pollen and foods, reducing pain in joints and muscles from inflammatory disorders and lessening joint deterioration; improves certain gastrointestinal ailments (such as stomach ulcers) and infections (such as candida); helps alleviate emphysema; and, since it's a component of insulin, helps diabetics. MSM is also well-known for strengthening brittle hair and nails, healing and strengthening damaged skin, and smoothing out wrinkles, due to its ability to help the body replace old, stiff skin cells with good healthy elastic cells. Indeed, I stumbled upon this much welcomed side effect myself when I started to take MSM regularly to tackle my body burden of mercury following the removal of my mercury fillings. I and other people noticed that my facial wrinkles markedly faded over time.

This nutrient is found in many foods, particularly fresh fruits and vegetables such as onions, garlic, and broccoli, and high-protein foods such as meats and beans. However, processing, storage, and cooking destroys essential MSM-sulfur, so most people tend to be deficient in this nutrient. Vegetarians are also more likely to become deficient in sulphur. MSM is very safe for most people, and any that is not used is just excreted from the body.

As with the above-mentioned amino acids, people with existing kidney or liver disease should consult their doctor before taking MSM-sulfur. Though sulfur itself is not toxic to our bodies, some people with difficulty detoxing can be highly allergic to relatives of sulfur such as sulfites and sulfa drugs. Sulfites are used as a food preservative and can trigger asthma and other allergic reactions in people who are sensitive. People with multiple chemical sensitivities and inflammatory bowel disease and autistic children may have problems in metabolizing the sulfur in MSM-sulfur, and sometimes even amino acids. If you think you might be allergic to sulfur-containing substances, you should avoid sulfur-containing compounds as a precaution.

Probiotics

Probiotic means "for life," derived from the Latin "pro" and the Greek "bio." This contrasts with *antibiotic,* which means "against life." The term *probiotics* is now generally used to describe the living, beneficial bacteria that support digestion as well as vaginal and urinary tract health. These bacteria promote the body's natural immunity, keep us healthy, keep levels of harmful bacteria low, and help our digestion.

Our gastrointestinal tract is home to more than four hundred different species of bacteria, most of them beneficial. This large quantity of working bacteria perform important functions in our bodies and keep us healthy by:

➤ Increasing the absorption of minerals and vitamins and improving digestion, especially of milk products.

➤ Improving our immune system by producing antimicrobial substances that deter various bad bacteria. (This is important because many debilitating and degenerative diseases begin in the intestinal tract.)
➤ Increasing the absorption of calcium, which is important in the prevention of osteoporosis.
➤ Producing B vitamins.
➤ Supporting healthy liver function.
➤ Normalizing bowel elimination problems and promoting regularity.
➤ Preventing intestinal tract infections like *Candida* and *Helicobacter pylori* (present in stomach ulcer conditions).
➤ Alleviating bowel wind, bloating, and belching.
➤ Assisting in cholesterol management.
➤ Protecting us against harmful bacteria, fungi, and viruses.

When there are not enough beneficial bacteria in the body, harmful bacteria are more likely to invade us, taking up residence on the lining of our intestinal tract, multiplying, and spreading over more and more intestinal area causing symptoms like bloating, bowel wind, indigestion, constipation, and diarrhea. Many things lower levels of good bacteria, particularly poor diets, chemical toxins, and certain pharmaceutical drugs, particularly antibiotics. Taking probiotic supplements such as lactobacillus acidophilus (which helps guard your small intestine) and bifidobacteria (which protects your large intestine) can help sustain good health.

Fiber

There are two types of fiber that are valuable in detoxing. The first is insoluble fiber, commonly referred to as roughage. Insoluble fiber, such as wheat bran, is not digested but passes though the gut unchanged. It is useful because it speeds the movement of waste products through the bowels—reducing the chance of the body reabsorbing toxic waste products.

The second and more important type is soluble fiber. This forms a gel-like consistency when combined with water and is found in higher levels in beans, seeds, oats, apples, and oranges. You can buy it in supplement form as ground-up psyllium seeds, fruit pectins, and gums. Also you should drink plenty of fluids with soluble fibers, in particular with psyllium husks, as they tend to absorb a lot of water.

These soluble fibers play an exceptionally important part in the Toxic Overload program because they are among the few substances that can lower the level of virtually all the different types of chemical toxins found in the body (such as organochlorines and toxic metals such as mercury). This is due to their powerful ability to bind themselves to dangerous toxins while traveling through the digestive system so that you can then excrete them safely.

Not only can these substances bind the most persistent chemicals in your body, but they also bind some of the essential nutrients that we need. When taking any fiber in the form of supplements, you should ideally take vitamins and minerals at least half an hour and preferably a whole hour after the soluble fiber. You can either take them once a day with your largest meal, or take smaller amounts before meals throughout the day. Furthermore, the binding substances in fiber can be so effective that they could potentially bind with any medications you are taking, thereby reducing their effect. So check with your doctor before taking a fiber supplement if you are on prescribed medications, particularly the contraceptive pill or thyroid hormone replacement treatment, as these could possibly be rendered ineffective.

The Daily Supplement Program

See "Daily Supplement Program" (p. 50) for the dosage requirements of the most important nutrients for chemical detox. You can take all the recommended supplements and essential fats in the morning. But

Daily Supplement Program

Multivitamin and mineral supplement: 1 per day (see "Levels of Vitamins and Minerals Desired in a Multivitamin," page 41)

Vitamin C: 500–2,000 mg (this is the total amount supplied from multivitamin and mineral preparation and separate supplementation)

Magnesium: 400–500 mg

Omega-3: 3–5 grams (1 tablespoon of flaxseed oil or 4–5 g purified fish oils should give you the optimum amount of omega-3 oils)

Amino Acids:
   Glutathione: 200–500 mg
   Cystine: 500–2,000 mg
   Taurine: 500–1,500 mg
   Methionine: 200–500 mg
   Or
   MSM-sulphur: 750–3,000 mg

Probiotics: Take as recommended on the container.

Soluble fiber supplement:

   Ground psyllium seeds and husks, or fruit pectin: 3–10 g (take before a meal with a large glass of water)
   Other sources of soluble fiber are also acceptable such as other fruit pectins, and guar and acacia gums.

if you can manage it, split the dose by taking some in the morning and some in the evening. A split dose is particularly useful for vitamin C, which lasts for only about eight hours in the body. If you take the total daily amount in two doses you will give your body better protection.

It is important not to take your supplements at the same time as soluble fiber. If you take the supplements and fiber too close together, the fiber may soak up some of these essential nutrients. Ideally, you should take the soluble fiber with some water as soon as you wake up in the morning, then by the time you have dressed and had breakfast you can take the supplements, but leave at least thirty minutes between the two, longer if possible. If you want to split the vitamin doses through the day, taking the soluble fiber before a meal and the supplements after a meal will allow sufficient time between doses. Alternatively, you could take the soluble fiber first thing in the morning, and take the supplements through the day.

CHAPTER 3

Step 2. Seven-Day Desludge Diet

STEP 2 REQUIRES MORE ATTENTION and will be an ongoing process, as it will take time to change your shopping habits and lifestyle accordingly. Be realistic about what you can achieve here. While it is very hard to eat and drink healthily all the time, the greater the proportion of beneficial foods in your diet, the better. In most cases, the primary way in which chemicals enter the body is through food, so you can avoid dangerous toxins by buying organic foods.

Chemicals in food originate from three main sources: pesticides and added chemicals, packaging and storage contamination, and environmental pollution. With the Seven-Day Desludge Diet, you will learn how to avoid these concentrated chemicals in your food and discover how to prepare and plan meals that will help you rid your system of these health damaging and often fattening toxins.

Pesticides and Added Chemicals

Conventional agriculture uses large amounts of pesticides, many of which are damaging to your health, to kill bugs and other pests and to stop food from spoiling. The foods containing the highest levels of pesticides tend to be perishable foods such as fresh fruits and vegetables, the majority of which contain one or more pesticides. Poultry and cattle farming use antibiotics to speed up growth, resulting in these chemicals ending up in the meat. Unfortunately, despite being contaminated by a host of chemicals such as fungicides (carbamates), insecticides (organophosphates), and antibiotics, none of the chemicals used in the growing of foods are listed on the food's label when you buy it in the store. So you simply cannot tell what chemical is likely to be on your strawberry or apple or in your steak. The best way to avoid pesticides in your foods is to buy organic produce and meat so that you can be sure that no toxic artificial chemicals were used in their production.

Fortunately, when chemicals are deliberately added to foods in the form of colorings and preservatives, the manufacturer is required to list these on the label. However, there are dozens of different additives on the market, and reading labels can be very confusing. The best way to avoid additives in foods is again to buy organic. Some foods that are not organic are also marked as having no artificial additives, preservatives, and colorings, and these are much healthier than regularly processed foods. In general, you should avoid foods with the following additives listed as ingredients on the label:

- ➤ Caffeine
- ➤ Bromate
- ➤ Olestra
- ➤ Hydrogenated vegetable oil
- ➤ Coloring known as blue 1, blue 2, green 3, red 3, or yellow 6
- ➤ Preservatives such as nitrate or sodium nitrate
- ➤ Flavoring known as monosodium glutamate
- ➤ All artificial sweeteners, particularly saccharine, aspartame, acesulfame K, and cyclamate potassium.

Did You Know?

More than one hundred pesticide ingredients are suspected to cause birth defects, cancer, and gene mutations.

More than 1 million children are exposed to unsafe levels of pesticides in their food.

Packaging and Storage Contamination

Before any food reaches your mouth, there are many ways in which chemicals can still sneak into it. Plastic or metal packaging, cooking containers, utensils, and food coverings can all contaminate food with toxic chemicals. The chemicals in plastic are highly fat soluble so any fatty foods placed in direct contact with a plastic will act like blotting paper and absorb the toxins directly from the plastic.

It can be a nightmare trying to avoid buying fatty foods in plastic containers, since they all seem to be wrapped in them. To minimize the extent of contamination from plastics, do not buy prewrapped foods and instead opt for foods stored in glass containers or made fresh at the deli. When you get them home, remove them from any temporary plastic wrappings and put them in natural containers such as glass, ceramic, cardboard, or paper. The longer the food is in contact with the plastic—and the higher the temperature of the food in the container—the greater the final level of food contamination. Do not heat up or place hot food in plastic or styrene containers, as it will greatly increase the level of contamination. Be particularly careful of carry-out food from restaurants, which is often placed hot in styrene containers.

Storing or buying salty, acidic, or high-fruit-content foods in aluminum containers (such as carbonated beverages in cans) can cause high levels of metal contamination. By transferring these foods to more natural alternatives such as glass, wood, metal (stainless steel is fine),

Did You Know?

A Swiss food scientist, Dr. Hans Hertel, found that microwave cooking alters a food's nutrients enough so that it can cause health-damaging changes in a person's blood, including:

➤ Increased cholesterol levels

➤ Increased levels of leukocytes (white blood cells), which suggests poisoning

➤ Decreased numbers of red blood cells

➤ Production of radiolytic compounds (compounds unknown in nature)

➤ Decreased hemoglobin levels, which could indicate anemic tendencies

or porcelain-based containers and cookware, you can ensure that you will not get a mouthful of health-damaging chemicals along with your food.

Environmental Pollutants

Fish and seafood can be heavily polluted with heavy metals and persistent toxins such as organochlorines (see chapter 1) because some parts of the sea are heavily polluted. Environmental pollution levels tend to be highest in animal fat, particularly if the animal or fish is a predator (such as salmon or tuna). Because organochlorines are highly fat-soluble chemicals, they are extremely persistent and they accumulate up the food chain. So if, for example, a salmon eats a smaller fish that carries a load of toxins, these toxins will be added to those already carried by the salmon.

Preparation and Storage Tips for Nonorganic Foods

➤   Peel the skin off of fresh fruits and vegetables.

➤   Thoroughly cook produce that does not have skin, such as broccoli and cauliflower.

➤   Eat low-fat animal products.

➤   Remove excess fat from meats and fish.

➤   Store food in glass and other nonplastic containers.

➤   Avoid consumption of foods prepackaged in plastic or aluminum containers or wrappings.

You can significantly reduce your dietary intake of deliberately added chemicals by buying organic foods, limiting your exposure to synthetic chemicals added during production, and peeling conventionally grown fruit and vegetables to reduce the levels of surface-borne chemicals. For vegetables you can't peel, such as broccoli, if you boil or cook them in water, most of the chemicals will be removed while cooking. Just be sure to discard the cooking water and do not use it for food preparation. Store food in glass, ceramic, or other nonplastic containers. Reduce your intake of seafood, particularly salmon and trout. Cut down your intake of animal fats, and substitute with vegetable oils.

The Benefits of Organic Foods

Organic foods are simply foods that are grown without most of the synthetic chemicals used in conventional farming, with a minimum level, if any, of synthetic pesticides, antibiotics, growth hormones, or fertilizers. Pretty much like the food humans were eating since time began, up to the

Beware of Genetically Modified Foods

For the past few years I have tried without success to find at least one study that has looked at the long-term effects on humans (or even animals) of eating genetically modified (GM) foods. I have found none. What is worse, in the few studies I have found, all on animals, each appeared to find some sort of short-term negative health effect, usually a shortening of life expectancy. The fact that genetically modified foods were originally treated by the Environmental Protection Agency (EPA) as a form of pesticide, and not food, suggests that the people registering them must have believed from the start that they would be potentially dangerous to our health.

One study conducted by researchers from the Norwegian Institute of Gene Ecology found that villagers living near a GM maize field in the Philippines have suffered a range of illnesses. Professor Terje Traavik, scientific director at Gen-Øk-Norwegian Institute of Gene Ecology, revealed details of a study showing that the villagers suffered fevers, breathing problems, and intestinal and skin ailments. He said blood tests indicated that the symptoms resulted from inhaling mutated maize pollen that had been carried in on the wind. The GM maize involved had been modified to include a pesticide called Bt within the plant.

Due to the increasing reports of toxicities from GM foods, the absence of even the most basic safety studies, and the fact that they have been treated as pesticides (and therefore actually designed to kill) and not foods, I would strongly recommend that all GM foods be avoided.

beginning of this century. This means that organically grown foods end up being lower in chemicals than their intensively grown counterparts.

Not only do organic foods have fewer deliberately added chemicals, but they also tend to be more resistant to being contaminated with environmentally acquired chemicals, such as heavy metals and organochlorines pollutants, owing to an increased resistance by way of growing in a more naturally nutritious and balanced soil or being fed a more nutritious and balanced diet.

In addition to an improved flavor and texture, organically grown foods also have an increased nutritional content, largely due to having been grown in better soil without artificial fertilizers. These multiple benefits are why I regularly buy organics for my family and strongly recommend them to anyone interested in their health.

Foods and Drinks to Avoid

There are some foods that you should definitely avoid on the Seven-Day Desludge Diet because they slow down or impair your ability to detoxify.

CAFFEINATED DRINKS

Caffeine is not a good substance to consume in large amounts because despite giving a temporary boost, it ultimately causes a decrease in energy. Not surprisingly, these low periods make you crave more caffeine to get back to the initial high. The continual fluctuation in energy hormones resulting from a high caffeine intake ends up causing a major disturbance and reduction in the level of energy-promoting and detoxing hormones. This brings with it strong carbohydrate cravings. In addition, caffeine also increases the rate at which the body loses many valuable and energy-giving nutrients such as magnesium, which can exacerbate the situation. As the decaffeinating process can itself be a source of chemicals, if you do drink decaffeinated coffee or tea, make sure that they have been decaffeinated using the natural Swiss water-decaffeination method.

ALCOHOL

Alcohol can slow down detoxification by slowing down our body's ability to process artificial chemicals, many of which also contain alcohol-like structures. They also use up a whole raft of nutrients, which are not only essential for powering the body, particularly the B group of vitamins, but are also essential in detoxifying the vast majority of toxic chemicals. This is why drinking alcohol when detoxing is not advised, and limiting alcohol at other times is the best way forward.

TRANS-FATS

Trans-fats are created when polyunsaturated oils and fats are heated in cooking. Food fried in sunflower oil, for example, is high in trans-fats; so is most deep-fried food. As these trans-fats not only prevent the uptake of good essential fats but also block their use in the body, they can lead to nutritional deficiencies. Limit yourself to cooking with olive oil, as it contains very little polyunsaturated fat.

Preparing for the Seven-Day Desludge Diet

This Seven-Day Desludge Diet is the next step to effective detoxing after starting the supplement program. It will help provide you with a highly effective way of getting your body's detox and health systems into shape. The foods I have included are great detoxers packed with lots of soluble fiber and bursting with essential detoxing and health-enhancing nutrients. Not only will this plan give your body the best start possible, if you continue some of these habits after having completed the initial Seven-Day Desludge Diet, you will be starting the rest of your life fully prepared to defend yourself from chemical-induced diseases.

While it is best to eat organic foods, for many it is not possible due to restricted availability or expense. The best advice is to avoid the most polluted foods (see page 60) and reduce the chemical loading of conventionally grown foods by peeling them, or by cutting excess fat off meat as most of the chemicals tend to be concentrated in the fat.

Below you will find a seven-day menu plan, which includes suggested times at which to take your supplements. This is a practical guide designed to make the whole program as easy as possible.

PROTEINS

You should eat at least 12 ounces (300 grams) of the following meats (preferably organic) or high-protein foods every day. Remove all visible

The Dirty Dozen

In my last book, *The Body Restoration Plan,* using nationally published and publicly available U.S. data, I calculated which foods were most contaminated with metabolism-blocking chemicals. In the number-one spot, as you can see, butter is the most contaminated food, with the others following in descending order:

1. Butter, salted
   (Unsalted butter has not been tested, but is likely to be contaminated as well.)
2. Salmon, steaks or fillets, fresh or frozen
3. Spinach, fresh or frozen
4. Strawberries, raw
5. Cream cheese
6. Raisins
7. Apple, red, raw, unpeeled
8. Dill cucumber pickles
9. Summer squash, fresh or frozen
10. Green peppers
11. Collards, fresh or frozen
12. Processed cheese

skin and fat from meat and fish when preparing them for cooking and don't eat the skin or fat on cooked meats. I have not included dairy products as a protein selection in this seven-day diet because large quantities could affect absorption of nutrients. In addition, many people appear to be intolerant of dairy products such as cheese and yogurts, which can exacerbate symptoms in a wide number of different diseases. There is an optional milk allowance, but while you are on the diet, dairy product intake should be restricted.

Healthy meat choices include:

➤ Lean beef or venison
➤ Chicken
➤ Turkey
➤ Vegetable-based proteins such as soy and Quorn (a high-protein, mushroom-based meat substitute)
➤ White fish (maximum of one fish meal every week)
➤ Eggs

OILS

In addition to the omega-3 supplement recommended in chapter 2, I recommend adding one of the following sources of healthy oils to your diet:

➤ 1 tablespoon of unprocessed vegetable oil such as walnut oil, pumpkin seed oil, or olive oil can be used cold in salads. It is best not to use oils other than olive oil in cooking as heating destroys their nutritional content.
➤ 1 ounce (28 grams) of raw nuts or raw seeds (or a combination) daily. Pumpkin seeds and walnuts are particularly healthful.
➤ 1 small avocado.

You can have an allowance of up to 4 fluid ounces (100 milliliters) of low-fat milk or unsweetened soymilk. The isoflavones in unsweetened soymilk are thought to help fight cancer, heart disease, high cholesterol, menopausal symptoms, and osteoporosis.

VEGETABLES

You can eat unlimited amounts of the following vegetables, raw, steamed, or as fat-free vegetable soup. Again, eat organic whenever possible.

➤ asparagus
➤ baby corn

- bamboo shoots
- beansprouts
- bell peppers; green, red, and yellow
- beets
- broccoli
- brussels sprouts
- cabbage
- carrots
- cauliflower
- celery
- Chinese cabbage
- cucumbers
- eggplant
- endive
- green beans
- green leafy vegetables
- leeks
- lettuce
- mange-tout (or sugar snap) peas
- mushrooms
- okra
- onions
- radishes
- Swiss chard
- tomatoes
- water chestnuts
- watercress
- zucchini

Raw Foods

The process of cooking lowers the levels of essential micronutrients in foods. As well as having a good micronutrient content, raw foods also contain a whole range of other nutrients, known as phytonutrients, which play a role in enhancing our body systems. Raw foods also have higher levels of the enzymes thought to improve digestion.

Drink Filtered Water

It is vitally important to drink water in sufficient quantities to help wash out toxins from the system. I would suggest an intake of at least two to three quarts (or liters) per day. Don't forget, if your body becomes mildly dehydrated by just a few percent, the level of energy you can produce will drop by 20 percent.

Tap water contains many chemicals that can enter the body either by the mouth or by being absorbed through the skin. As well as chlorine, water may be contaminated with other chemicals such as aluminum (deliberately added during processing), lead and plastics (from piping), and environmental pollution (pesticides in agricultural areas). A sink-top or whole-house water filter will significantly lower the levels of chemicals in tap water. Bottled water also tends to be less polluted than tap water, particularly if stored in glass.

Always filter or distill tap water before drinking it. If you use bottled water, buy it in a glass bottle in preference to a plastic one. If you can, install a household water filter to reduce the chemicals absorbed through the skin during baths and showers.

Soluble Fiber–Rich Foods

In addition to the fiber supplement recommended in chapter 2, you should ensure that your diet contains foods rich in soluble fiber such as:

➤ 6 ounces (160 grams) of cooked legumes such as lentils, split peas, kidney beans, peas (could be eaten raw), chickpeas, or green beans
➤ 2 ounces (50 grams) of oats
➤ 4 small oatcakes

Fruit

Eat four portions of fresh fruit a day. A typical portion of fruit is: an apple, an orange, half a grapefruit, two medium plums, a nectarine, a peach, a small banana, or 100 grams of any other fruit.

Beverages

Drink at least eight large glasses (225 milliliters) of freshly filtered or bottled water a day. As well as keeping you well hydrated, drinking plenty of water will also help flush away unwanted chemicals. To aid detoxification even more, drink mineral water and flavor it with lemon or lime juice. Caffeinated coffee or tea should be avoided on the seven-day detox, while coffee substitutes, herbal teas, and filtered water can be drunk freely. Drinks or other products using artificial sweeteners should be avoided.

Flavorings

The following flavorings can be used at anytime, and many of these, including fresh herbs, garlic, and yeast extracts, are very beneficial!

➤ herbs
➤ spices
➤ mustard
➤ chiles
➤ garlic
➤ pepper
➤ salt
➤ soy sauce
➤ lemon juice
➤ vinegar
➤ Worcestershire sauce
➤ yeast extracts
➤ bouillon cubes

The Seven-Day Desludge Diet

Day 1

Early morning	Fiber supplements Large glass of water
Breakfast	Tofu scramble: sauté tofu, diced onion, and herbs in 1 teaspoon of olive oil. Multivitamin and mineral supplement, magnesium, vitamin C, MSM-sulfur or amino acids, probiotics, and 1 tablespoon of flaxseed oil or pollution-free fish oil supplements (taken at least half an hour after fiber supplements)
Mid-morning	1 portion of fruit
Pre-lunch	Fiber supplements Large glass of water
Lunch	Chicken, apple, and beet salad with red leaf lettuce topped with a teaspoon of sliced raw almonds
Afternoon	Two plums
Pre-dinner	Fiber supplements Large glass of water
Dinner	Roast beef or grilled beef steak Curried chickpeas: slice an onion, garlic, chili pepper, and zucchini. Sauté in 1 teaspoon of olive oil until soft, then add a small can of chopped tomatoes and 5 ounces of cooked chickpeas and cook for 5 to 10 minutes. Flavor with pinch of salt and pepper, garam masala, and cumin seeds (ground or whole). Add chopped fresh coriander and serve. A slice of melon

Day 2

Early morning   Fiber supplements
Large glass of water

Breakfast   Oatmeal (made with water and with milk from allowance, see page 61.)
Multivitamin and mineral supplement, magnesium, vitamin C, MSM-sulfur or amino acids, probiotics, and 1 tablespoon of flaxseed oil or pollution-free fish oil supplements (taken at least half an hour after fiber supplements)

Mid-morning   1 portion of fruit

Pre-lunch   Fiber supplements
Large glass of water

Lunch   Roast chicken deli chicken breast
Mixed salad with red and green bell peppers and unlimited vegetables, dressed with lemon juice and herbs
1 orange

Afternoon   1 portion of fruit

Pre-dinner   Fiber supplements
Large glass of water

Dinner   Grilled steak
Steamed green beans
Apple, 1 ounce (28 grams) of walnuts, and green salad, dressed with lemon juice
Any additional supplements

Day 3

Early morning	Fiber supplements Large glass of water
Breakfast	Banana and mango smoothie Two oatcakes Multivitamin and mineral supplement, magnesium, vitamin C, MSM-sulfur or amino acids, probiotics, and 1 tablespoon of flaxseed oil or pollution-free fish oil supplements (taken at least half an hour after fiber supplements)
Mid-morning	Cucumber and raw vegetable sticks
Pre-lunch	Fiber supplements Large glass of water
Lunch	Grilled or steamed white fish Steamed broccoli and carrots 2 oatcakes
Afternoon	1 portion of fruit
Pre-dinner	Fiber supplements Large glass of water
Dinner	Beef, green pepper, and onion kebabs Mediterranean salad of sliced tomato, cucumber, and avocado with a sprinkling of coriander and olives 1 portion of fruit Any additional supplements

Day 4

Early morning   Fiber supplements
Large glass of water

Breakfast   2 eggs: scramble with herbs and tomatoes in 1 teaspoon of olive oil.
1 small glass of freshly squeezed orange juice
Multivitamin and mineral supplement, magnesium, vitamin C, MSM-sulfur or amino acids, probiotics
and 1 tablespoon of flaxseed oil or pollution-free fish
oil supplements (taken at least half an hour after fiber
supplements)

Mid-morning   1 portion of fruit

Pre-lunch   Fiber supplements
Large glass of water

Lunch   Lean deli meat
White bean, tomato, lettuce, and onion salad
dressed with lemon juice and seasoned with salt and
pepper.

Afternoon   1 portion of fruit

Pre-dinner   Fiber supplements
Large glass of water

Dinner   1 slice of melon
Spicy tofu: stirfry using seasoned tofu, garlic, onions,
mushrooms, chiles, red peppers, zucchini, tomatoes,
and 2 teaspoons of olive oil.
Any additional supplements

Day 5

Early morning   Fiber supplements
Large glass of water

Breakfast   Sugar-free muesli topped with a sliced banana
Multivitamin and mineral supplement, magnesium, vitamin C, MSM-sulfur or amino acids, probiotics, and 1 tablespoon of flaxseed oil or pollution-free fish oil supplements (taken at least half an hour after fiber supplements)

Mid-morning   1 apple

Pre-lunch   Fiber supplements
Large glass of water

Lunch   Turkey burger
Orange, raw grated carrot, 1 ounce (28 grams) of raw pumpkin seeds, and green leaf salad dressed with lemon juice

Afternoon   1 portion of fruit

Pre-dinner   Fiber supplements
Large glass of water

Dinner   Consommé or clear soup broth
Grilled chicken breast
Steamed leeks and mushrooms with tomato sauce
Fresh fruit salad
Any additional supplements

Day 6

Early morning   Fiber supplements
Large glass of water

Breakfast   Oatmeal (made with water and milk from allowance, see page 61.)
Multivitamin and mineral supplement, magnesium, vitamin C, MSM-sulfur or amino acids, probiotics, and 1 tablespoon of flaxseed oil or pollution-free fish oil supplements (taken at least half an hour after fiber supplements)

Mid-morning   Small bunch of grapes

Pre-lunch   Fiber supplements
Large glass of water

Lunch   Warm turkey, roast garlic, spinach, and pine nut salad: Roast 4 cloves of garlic for about 15 minutes in 1 teaspoon of olive oil until slightly brown. Immediately mix with warmed pieces of turkey and arrange over baby spinach leaves, then sprinkle with a teaspoon of pine nuts and flavor with lemon juice, salt, and pepper.
1 banana

Afternoon   1 portion of fruit

Pre-dinner   Fiber supplements
Large glass of water

Dinner   Grilled beef steak
Vegetable bake: Slice tomatoes, zucchini, yellow bell pepper, mushrooms, and garlic, then brush with olive oil and bake until vegetables are tender.
1 pear
Any additional supplements

Day 7

Early morning	Fiber supplements Large glass of water
Breakfast	Banana and pineapple smoothie 2 oat cakes Multivitamin and mineral supplement, magnesium, vitamin C, MSM-sulfur or amino acids, probiotics, and 1 tablespoon of flaxseed oil or pollution-free fish oil supplements (taken at least half an hour after fiber supplements)
Mid-morning	Raw carrot and cucumber sticks
Pre-lunch	Fiber supplements Large glass of water
Lunch	Grilled chicken breast Mixed green leaf and herb salad: In a large bowl, mix salad and chopped fresh herbs, add cherry tomatoes, dress with lemon juice and 1 tablespoon of olive oil. Season with salt and pepper and serve.
Afternoon	1 apple and 2 oatcakes
Pre-dinner	Fiber supplements Large glass of water
Dinner	1 slice of melon Grilled white fish Braised or steamed mange-tout (or sugar snap) peas, baby corn, and carrots Any additional supplements

CHAPTER 4

Step 3. Chemical-Free Home and Beauty Products

NOT ONLY ARE WE SUBJECTED to a barrage of chemicals in our food, we also are breathing them in every time we clean our house, and are smothering ourselves with them every time we put on suntan lotion, face or body creams, or the many other beauty products available. While it is virtually impossible to cut chemicals out of your life entirely, it is possible to dramatically slash the amount that gets through by paying attention to the products you use to furnish and clean your house and those that you put on your face and body.

Many toxic chemicals are commonly found in building materials, fabrics, and furnishings. The average room has many potential hot spots. The key to successfully reducing the amount of toxins in your home is not to completely renovate it, but to attempt to furnish your home with materials made from natural, untreated fabrics and materials when replacing old furnishings and fittings. You also need to detox it by removing existing concentrated sources of chemicals, and stop re-polluting it with poisonous cleaning preparations. While it can take a bit of getting used to, any efforts you make to lower your overall exposure to chemicals in your home and garden will be repaid in better health and a higher level of energy.

Did You Know?

Indoor levels of pollutants may be two to five times—and occasionally more than 1,000 times—higher than outdoor levels.

The rest of the information in this chapter will help you detoxify your home and life by showing you how to remove typical toxins from your home and garden. Once you know where the highest concentrated sources of chemicals can be located, it will be possible to convert even the most polluted home into a safe, relaxing, low-chemical oasis. Then, you will learn how to treat your body to clean and rejuvenating beauty products that will limit your exposure to many common toxins.

Sources of Chemicals in a Typical Room

Most chemicals that contaminate the home stem from the use of the following groups of substances:

➤ Pesticides in pest-control products (such as roach and flea treatments), wood treated for dry rot, mothproofing in wool carpets, paints, air pollution, and contaminated water.
➤ Plastics and plasticizers in household fittings and ornaments, children's toys, computers, air fresheners, polluted air, carpet treatments, vinyl flooring, any PVC product, dust contaminants, paints, wallpaper (many wallpapers are actually vinyl) and wallpaper adhesives, curtain fabrics, and carpets and underlay.
➤ Flame retardants in many fabrics and upholstery.
➤ Solvents in carpets, fiberboard, chipboard, paints, air fresheners, finishes, cleaning solutions, office corrective fluids, cosmetics, polluted air, and glues.

➤ Lead and dust from peeling and chipped paint, and water stored in or flowing through lead pipes.

Pest-Control Products

Virtually every kitchen has a "killing corner," a cupboard or shelf that is filled to the brim with all kinds of fly and roach sprays, insect repellents, flea powders and shampoos, and a battery of other deadly synthetic chemicals. These products not only contain "active" pesticides, but sometimes more than 99 percent of their contents are ingredients that have been classified as "inert," which, though it sounds harmless, can include deadly, cancer-causing, highly toxic substances such as formaldehyde, analine, benzene, and the toxic metals lead, cadmium, and even mercury. These chemicals are used in pesticide products to increase efficiency and make them easier to use.

The health effects of exposure to these pesticide products range from mild to severe and may include dizziness, nausea, acute poisoning, cancer, neurological effects, and reproductive and developmental harm. In many cases, effects are not immediate and may show up years later as unexplained illness.

However, due to their "protected" status (for financial reasons) and despite the extremely well-documented toxicity of many of them, inert substances don't have to be listed on a product's label. Furthermore, government officials are forbidden by law from revealing the inert ingredients in pesticide products. While manufacturers are required to provide the Environmental Protection Agency (EPA) with names of all pesticide ingredients including inerts, the EPA routinely withholds this information from the public because of industry claims that the information is subject to trade secrecy laws.

By law, the EPA is prohibited from disclosing confidential business information (CBI) to the public. However, the agency may disclose CBI in limited circumstances, such as when necessary to treat illness or injury or to prevent imminent harm to people, property, or the environment. Even then, release of the information must often be limited to certain

Chemical-Free Pest Control Tips

Remove all food waste from the kitchen every night to discourage potential pests from making your home theirs. There are also many natural products you can make at home or get at any health food store to rid your kitchen and home of most bugs and pests.

➤   Deodorize your kitchen with a room spray made of water and a few drops of essential citrus oils.

➤   Eliminate cockroaches with a powder made of equal parts baking soda and powdered sugar. Spread this mixture where they congregate and repeat every one to two weeks until they are gone.

➤   Wipe out ants by mixing one cup of water with two teaspoons of essential peppermint oil and spray the mixture wherever the ants come in—on windowsills, countertops, and along skirting boards.

➤   Get rid of your cat's or dog's fleas by using an herbal shampoo, spray, or flea collar, all of which contain natural repellents such as pennyroyal or eucalyptus oil. There are even herbal flea powders to use on carpets and furnishings. They usually contain pyrethrum (a plant extract) or borax.

"qualified persons" such as medical personnel, who may not disseminate the information more broadly.

Since the majority of ingredients in many pesticide products are so-called inerts—up to 99 percent in some cases—this is a significant issue. According to the National Coalition Against the Misuse of Pesticides (NCAMP), there are more than 2,300 inert substances added to pesticide products. The EPA has reportedly conceded that it does not have the information to assess the toxicity of more than three-quarters of the chemicals used as inerts.

These products should all be banished from your kitchen and your house because of the real health risk they pose to you and your family. But don't put them down the sink where they will poison the water supply—dispose of them responsibly by taking them to an authorized municipal dump.

Cleaning Products

The vast majority of domestic cleaning products contain an abundance of toxic chemicals, most of which could seriously impact your health. Indeed, household cleansers are the major source of home toxins. Approximately 500,000 tons of liquid cleaners are washed down U.S. drains annually. These products are absorbed through the skin, breathed into the lungs, and eaten from plates with chemical residue following "cleaning." Ingestion, of course, is always a danger as well, and the number-one cause of household poisoning is dish detergent.

Most cleaning products rely on petroleum-based surfactants, solvents, and other chemicals, some of which are known to be acutely toxic in large doses. Others have been linked to reproductive illnesses and cancer. Most of these chemicals have not been tested for their impact on human health. Many household cleansers contain substances such as the highly toxic halogens chlorine and fluorine as well as glycol ether, naphtha, and kerosene, which are neurotoxins and central-nervous-system depressants. These substances can cause confusion, headaches, lack of concentration, and symptoms of mental illness.

Some of these products contain such a toxic cocktail of chemicals that the EPA has produced guides to help people choose environmentally friendly chemicals and avoid products that contain the following seventeen highly toxic substances: benzene, cadmium, carbontetrachloride, chloroform, cyanide, lead, mercury, dichloromethane, chromium, methyl ethyl ketone, methyl isobutyl ketone, nickel, tetrachloroethylene, 1,1,1-trichloroethane, toluene, trichloroethylene, and xylenes.

Other chemicals commonly found in cleaning products are surfactants—substances that remove fat, proteins, and dust from clothes or surfaces to ensure that the fats and dirt dissolve in the washing water without sticking to the clothes or surface again. Many ordinary household products such as detergents, cleaning agents, dishwashing liquids, soaps, shampoos, and conditioners contain surfactants. These chemicals are well known to be toxic to fish and in aquatic systems. The toxicity of these surfactants on humans varies, but in many cases they can cause severe skin, eye, and respiratory harm. What's more, when surfactants, which are classified as "inert" pesticide additives, are mixed with other active chemicals, they can hugely increase the toxicity of other chemicals—whether toxic chemicals in cleaning solutions or "active" pesticides in pest-control preparations.

The best thing to do is to clear them all out, and try to find healthier alternatives. To be honest, despite the continuing media hype, cleaning a home doesn't require specialized and expensive ingredients. All you really need is white vinegar, lemon juice, baking soda, and/or borax diluted with water to make a liquid or paste. All of these mixtures make cheap and safe cleaning products. If you don't want to make your own cleaning solutions, you'll find plenty of alternative, environmentally friendly cleaning products in your local health food store or supermarket. One brand of nontoxic cleaning supplies is Ecover, and I use their products for virtually all my cleaning needs, from laundry

Did You Know?

➤ An EPA study revealed that toxic chemicals in household cleaners are three times more likely to cause cancer than outdoor air.

➤ The Asthma Society of Canada has identified common household cleaners and cosmetics as triggers to asthma.

soap to dishwasher tablets. The next time you run out of one product or another, whether it's floor cleaner, window cleaner, or bathroom cleaner, replace it with something less harmful.

If there are particular products you really can't find a replacement for, seal them up in an airtight container such as a tin after each use. This will significantly reduce the amount of vapor they release into the air, which would otherwise end up in your lungs. While vapor will escape when you open the tin container, it will not continually contaminate your environment as it would if left out in its original container.

Carpets

All carpets, whether synthetic or wool, are known to gather and hold a large quantity of household dust and to act as sanctuaries for a large quantity of toxic chemicals. In particular, household pesticide residues may not stay where they are applied, and after application in the home, some pesticides can vaporize from solid to gas and redeposit them-

Chemical-Free Cleaning Tips

➤ Use a mixture of white vinegar and water to clean windows.

➤ Prepare a mixture of lemon juice and water to wash your dishes, clean your bathroom, and wipe down counters.

➤ Dilute baking soda or borax in water to create a scrubbing cleanser.

➤ Purchase environmentally friendly cleaning products at your local health food store (see Resources for specific product recommendations).

➤ Store your chemical-laden cleaning products in airtight containers.

selves throughout the home—on carpets, floors, bedding, even children's toys. Carpets, furniture, and house dust have been identified as long-term reservoirs for pesticides, and residues of some pesticides persist in carpets for up to a year. One study detected a greater number of pesticides in carpet dust than were found in the air of individual homes. Preliminary data show that children in contact with household surfaces treated with insecticides absorb two to fifteen times more chemicals than their parents.

Carpets in older houses that still contain lead-based paints can also have seriously dangerous levels of lead dust due to years of accumulation. These dusts are so fine that normal vacuuming can actually make the problem worse by dispersing them into the air. Specialized vacuums containing HEPA (high efficiency particle absorption) filters should be used to remove lead dust. However, if lead detection specialists find lead dust levels to be exceedingly high, it is probably better to remove the whole carpet using the correct protocol as reported by the U.S. Environmental Protection Agency (1994) in their pamphlet *Reducing Lead Hazards When Remodeling Your Home* (Washington, D.C., Office of Pollution Prevention and Toxics, EPA 747-R-94-002). If the correct method is not used, large amounts of lead could be released into the air.

Synthetic carpets are themselves made from dozens of toxic chemicals, such as benzene, formaldehyde, and styrene. They can also contain up to 120 carcinogenic chemicals (including installation materials). Symptoms reported to the Consumer Product Safety Commission (CPSC) from being exposed to synthetic carpets include burning eyes, memory problems, chills and fevers, sore throats, chest tightness, cough, numbness, depression, and difficulty concentrating. The EPA considers synthetic carpet to be a major contributor of volatile organic compounds to indoor air pollution and has safety information available for consumers. What's more, in 1991, the attorneys general of twenty-six states petitioned the CPSC to require health warnings on new carpet and installation materials, but the CPSC refused, saying the action was "premature."

You may be surprised to discover that a natural product such as wool carpet can often contain more toxic chemicals than some synthetic carpets. This is due to the fact that all manufacturers have to use pesticides to mothproof the wool and carpet backing. Even the underlay contains chemicals from the plastics and other solvents used in their manufacture.

Using many of the widely available carpet "cleaning" or stain removing products only adds to the chemical load of your carpet. Most ordinary carpet cleaners and spot removers contain an unhealthy concoction of toxic chemicals, such as formaldehyde, solvents, acids, heavy metals, pesticides, disinfectants, synthetic fragrances, and many others. Fabric and carpet stain repellents or "guards" may contain plastics and have a history of containing organofluorines, powerful hormone disruptors, and accumulate in the tissues of humans. During application and drying, the chemicals in these carpet products evaporate and may concentrate in the air, causing indoor air pollution, especially if the room is not well ventilated.

Carpet shampoos generally contain solvents and detergents that must be applied for a specific period of time and then vacuumed to remove the product. A residue may be left behind or the product may sink deep enough into carpets so that they cannot be pulled out by the vacuum cleaner. Powders or dusts are easily inhaled and may irritate airways or cause asthma attacks. In fact, anti–dust mite carpet treatments sometimes contain tannic acid or the common preservative benzyl benzoate, both of which are skin, eye, and lung irritants. Deodorizing powders often contain fragrances that irritate asthmatic lungs as well.

Did You Know?

Synthetic carpets can contain cancer-causing chemicals such as benzene, formaldehyde, and styrene, as well as toxins that affect the central nervous system.

Indoor air pollution caused by chemicals in carpet cleaning products can cause headaches, irritation to eyes, nose, and lungs, congestion, sneezing, coughing, fatigue, nausea, and other symptoms. Long-term exposure to carpet cleaners may increase the risks for chronic illnesses such as heart disease and cancer, depending on the chemicals involved. There is also evidence of a link between carpet cleaners and Kawasaki disease. This is a childhood disease, mainly affecting those aged one to five years old, which can damage heart blood vessels and increase the risk for cardiac thrombosis (heart attack). This link is particularly strong when children are exposed to carpet cleaning fumes within four hours of application.

So what's the alternative? Organic carpet is becoming more widely available, and, unlike virtually every other carpet on the market, it won't come with these unwanted chemical extras. Another option is to try to source natural fiber carpets with jute backings that have not been treated with pesticides or other chemicals. You could also simply try to limit the amount of carpet in your home. Not only are washable throw rugs, tile, wood, and other noncarpet materials free of most of the toxins found in carpeting and carpet cleaners, they are also easier to keep clean.

The best carpet deodorizer is baking soda, as it soaks up odors instead of masking them. Sprinkle baking soda over the surface of the carpet. Let it stand for 15 to 30 minutes, or a few hours, even overnight, for stronger odors. Sweep up the larger amounts of baking soda, then vacuum the rest. Repeat the process if you still smell odors you wish to remove.

Baking soda works like magic, it sometimes just takes time and making sure you are using enough. Keep kids away so they don't inhale the baking soda while it's applied. Sweep up the larger amounts of baking soda, and vacuum up the rest. (Note that your vacuum cleaner bag will get full and heavy.) Caution: While damp baking soda works well to remove many odors, it can also get stuck onto the carpet fibers and be difficult to clean. If you live in a very humid climate and worry that the baking soda may become damp once applied, you might substitute a light spray of white distilled vinegar for the baking soda.

Chemical-Free Carpets

➤ Limit the amount of carpeting in your home as much as possible.

➤ Steam clean your carpets every 6 months either professionally or with a steamer rented from your local hardware store.

➤ Clean your carpets with a mixture of 1 cup of white vinegar and 2½ gallons of water (add another cup of vinegar for a stronger solution).

➤ If you must use soap or detergent, use a mixture of no more than 3–4 tablespoons of mild liquid soap or detergent and at least one gallon of water.

➤ Place doormats at all entrances.

➤ Encourage family members to remove shoes when coming in the home (this also prevents pesticides, pollutants, and dirt being tracked onto your carpet).

➤ Vacuum two or more times per week, particularly in high-traffic areas.

➤ Remove carpet stains by using a mixture of a few teaspoons of white vinegar and one cup of water. Let sit for several minutes then blot with another clean towel.

➤ If you live in a pre-1978 home and there are lead paints in your walls or woodwork, contact your local government authority about getting a specialist to test for lead dust in your carpet. You may need to have your carpet cleaned by a specialist or have it removed entirely.

Air Your Air

Airborne chemicals pose one of the greatest contamination threats in the home. These chemicals include lead, organochlorines (such as PCBs, dioxins), pesticides, asbestos, and plasticizers (such as phtalates). The largest amount of chemicals in the home comes from the hundreds of volatile solvents, or VOCs (such as formaldehyde), which are released from paint cans, cleaning solutions, carpets, and underlay.

The simplest and quickest way of ventilating your house and removing chemicals in the air is to simply open your windows. Try to make sure that you open windows at the front and back of the house, as this will increase the flow of air. This is particularly valuable in new houses, as many of them are now hermetically sealed to conserve energy. Ventilating the house for just half an hour a day can really make all the difference. Even if you live in a city, indoor air still tends to be far more polluted than city air, so it is still a good idea to allow some ventilation. Of course, if you live next to a very busy road it would be wise to close the windows during peak traffic hours. If the outside air is exceptionally polluted, you could always consider investing in an air filter, which can clean the air of chemicals from exhaust fumes.

Chemical-Free Ventilation Tips

➤ Open the windows in your home for at least half an hour a day.

➤ Place a plant in each room of your home. Plants that are particularly helpful in absorbing solvents from the atmosphere include spider plants, Boston ferns, elephant-ear philodendron, English ivy, and aloe vera.

Bedroom Toxins

The bedroom is a particularly important room, as most of us spend over one third of our lives there. Consequently, if any room needs to be free of chemicals this is the one. The easiest and most effective way to detoxify this room is simply to keep your window open at night.

Because of current fire regulations, most mattresses are now covered with flame retardants, which can constantly emit health-damaging formaldehyde gas and may contain brominated substances (see next paragraph). Today's modern beds are constructed from a wide range of petrochemical products such as vinyl and polyurethane foam. The latest research shows the petroleum chemicals used to make these materials are being emitted into your breathing zone while you sleep. The flexible polyurethane foam used in upholstered furniture, for example, can be up to 30 percent flame-retardant by weight.

We now know that brominated flame retardants escape from these products into our homes and the environment—and that they're building up at alarming rates in our bodies. New studies are showing serious health effects ranging from interference with prenatal brain development to disruption of hormone function and cancer. Since the chemicals found are known carcinogens and respiratory irritants, parents of children with cancer or asthma should be particularly concerned.

The closet or wardrobe tends to be the other major source of chemicals in the bedroom. Some will originate from clothes that contain plastics, such as synthetic leather or waterproofed clothing. Many fabrics receive a variety of chemical treatments to make them static-resistant, wrinkle-resistant, and flame-retardant. All children's sleepwear is required by law to meet federal flammability standards. Most fabrics treated with flame-retardant chemicals continuously emit toxic formaldehyde gas. Breathing formaldehyde gas above the levels of 0.1 parts per million for an extended period of time will cause many health problems, such as headaches, dizziness, scratchy eyes and throat, nasal congestion, coughing, and immune system abnormalities. Formalde-

Chemical-Free Bedroom Tips

➤ Put a hypo-allergenic mattress cover or an extra layer of blankets on your mattress. You can also buy an organic mattress.

➤ Use pillows filled with natural fibers such as cotton, wool, or feathers.

➤ Instead of mothballs, make sachets of potpourri that include natural lavender oil to hang in your closet.

➤ Buy clothes made of machine-washable, natural fibers as opposed to dry-clean-only clothes.

➤ If you must dry clean your clothes, air them out in a well-ventilated space for at least three days after cleaning, or find a dry cleaner that uses steam instead of chemicals for cleaning.

➤ Do not buy clothes with flame retardants in them for yourself or your family, except for infants and small children.

➤ Steer clear of purchasing products with chemical finishes, such as permanent press, wrinkle resistant, anti-static, and water or stain repellent.

➤ Avoid fabrics that have been treated with formaldehyde-based resins that can cause allergic skin reactions.

➤ Wash and dry all new clothing and bedding three times prior to using for the first time.

hyde resins can also cause similar symptoms. Unfortunately, most fabrics treated with flame-resistant chemicals continuously emit toxic and allergic formaldehyde gas at rates as high as 500 parts per million at the surface of the fabric.

You may even be responsible for adding to the chemical load in your clothes yourself if you have them dry cleaned (because of the solvents used in cleaning) or if you use certain chemically treated mothballs to prevent insect damage.

What's in Your Workroom or Office?

Unlike most people, those working with chemicals—cleaners, painters and decorators, car mechanics, and chemical factory workers—tend to get their greatest overall levels of chemicals from their work environment. These chemicals commonly consist of solvents, pesticides, toxic metals, and plasticizers, which can be breathed into the lungs or spread on the skin where they are then absorbed into the body. Although the levels entering via the skin and lungs tend to be lower than dietary levels, chemicals ingested in this way can be more toxic. This is because they have effectively bypassed the digestive system, which is normally responsible for breaking certain chemicals down, and have gone straight into the bloodstream. Since most of us spend so much of our lives at work, we need to see to it that our exposure to chemicals at work is as low as possible.

As with your home, you need to have good ventilation, particularly if you work with chemicals. And if the chemicals used to clean the office are overpowering, find out whether they can be used more sparingly (a good argument, as this will save your employer money) or replaced with natural products. It may also be a good idea to find out more about whether any pesticides are regularly sprayed in the building or discover more about the chemicals you are working with.

Nearly all workers today are exposed to some sort of chemical hazard, since chemicals are used in every type of industry. Therefore, whether you are a dental hygienist, cleaner, pest controller, beautician, or painter, it is important to learn as much as possible about the chemicals you work with. Ask to see the Material Safety Data Sheets if you work in the U.S., or contact the Workplace Hazardous Materials Information System (WHMIS) if you work in Canada for relevant information about the toxic chemicals found in products used in your workplace. You could insist on appropriate measures to control chem-

A Chemical-Free Work Environment

➤ Keep inks, carbon paper, liquid paper, and rubber cement in sealed containers.

➤ Place a plant in your office.

➤ Use the appropriate protective equipment whenever it is available, especially if working with hazardous chemicals.

➤ Find out as much as possible about the health hazards and the appropriate safety handling procedures of the chemicals you work with.

➤ Ensure good ventilation in your workplace.

➤ Don't bring your workplace chemicals home with you. If you work with chemicals, you should shower and change your clothes, before you leave work if necessary.

➤ If you work with chemicals, don't wash your work clothes with the family wash. Although you may think that the amount of chemical contaminant you bring home on your clothes (or skin) is small, over time this can add up to a significant exposure that could lead to a serious illness.

ical hazards, such as replacing toxic chemicals with less harmful substances, improving local exhaust ventilation, using personal protective equipment such as gloves, and using proper protective procedures for handling chemicals.

Home Renovations

When setting out on a home renovation project, you have to think about the type of new products to buy, since many new building materials can significantly pollute your house and seriously add to your chemical burden and risk of a wide range of diseases. Fumes from new decorating products like paint, carpets, and vinyl or pressed wood contribute to indoor air pollution, which is ranked among the top four environmental health risks by the EPA. As you renovate, microscopic particles and invisible gases can accumulate undetected in your home until they result in ill-effects such as burning of the eyes, nose, and throat, headaches, dizziness, fatigue, asthma attacks, and cold or hay-fever symptoms.

When renovating your home, it is important to know whether the materials you are discarding in your home are made of toxic substances which need to be handled carefully. Lead-based paints, lead pipes, and asbestos were all commonly used building materials in homes which are now banned, but which may still remain in your home and provide a significant health risk—especially when you are attempting to remove them as part of a home renovation project. You also need to be sure that the new materials you use will not emit dangerous fumes or cause a serious health risk in your home environment.

By knowing which chemicals are found where, it becomes possible to avoid them or deal with them safely so damage to you and your family's health can be minimized on any building project. Before starting on any building project, or even before buying an older house, request an environmental assessment to see if your home contains old lead paint or pipes, vinyl, pressed-wood surfaces, or asbestos insulation, in addition to previous use of wood treatments and other wood preservatives such as lindane. It is so important to know about the possible presence of these substances, because, if you don't, there is a risk of releasing large amounts of very hazardous substances into your home when building work starts. For instance, knocking down a wall or stripping it of old lead paint without carrying out certain precautions could release dangerous amounts of lead dust into your home.

A good company that provides environmental assessments is Environmental Construction Outfitters (ECO), which is based in New York (www.environproducts.com). Not only can they test your home for toxic substances but they also sell environmentally friendly, toxic-chemical-free building materials. There are many nontoxic alternatives available and many companies, such as the Environmental Home Center (www.built-e.com), BuildingGreen.com, and the Building for Health Materials Center (www.buildingforhealth.com), specialize in this area. As well as providing a fabulous source of information, these companies should help you to source low-chemical versions of virtually every thing you will ever need. Better still, in many cases the environmentally friendly option is not more expensive, and in some cases can actually be much cheaper. So be sure to ask whatever builder you use to use suppliers that provide environmentally-friendly products.

LEAD-BASED PAINT

While lead paints were banned in 1978, 38 million homes still have it on the walls. This may explain why one in six children—or nearly one million kids under the age of six in the U.S.—have worrisome levels of lead in their blood. Lead, a heavy metal, is a highly noxious neurotoxin. Lead poisoning in children can cause lowered IQ, memory loss, learning disabilities, impaired hearing, reduced attention spans, aggression, and other behavior problems. Children's risk usually is greatest in their earliest years because their brains are still developing. They are also at that explorative age when their curiosity may lead them to putting paint chips in their mouths.

If lead is found, but the paint is still intact (not chipping or peeling), then your family is safe from lead poisoning, but you will still need to have it removed from your home. If the lead paint is falling apart or was used on doorjambs or window frames, where constant movement and friction cause a dust to escape, you will need to take action because activities like opening a window or door coated with lead paint can create enough lead dust over time to harm a child.

A lead abatement specialist (see below) must clean up all lead paint. Do not attempt this yourself! The U.S. Department of Housing and Urban Development (HUD) or the American Industrial Hygiene Association can help you locate certified lead removal contractors in your area. As a temporary measure until lead paint is removed, damp mop frequently, particularly around areas of friction and increased wear and tear of lead-based paintwork, such as window frames or painted drawers. Also, wash surfaces with a bucket of phosphate-containing detergent solution (as this helps bind the lead) and then squeeze the dirty water into an empty bucket. This is known as the three-bucket cleaning system. Be sure to wash children's toys and stuffed animals frequently. Rent or buy a vacuum with a HEPA filter to remove lead dust. If possible, your family should move out while lead-based paint is being removed by a lead abatement professional.

PIPES

The second most common source of lead comes from lead pipes or lead-soldered copper pipes. Even though lead pipes are no longer sold or placed in new homes, they may still exist in older homes. Lead pipes were used in houses built before the 1920s, and also served as water mains connecting to homes. Lead solder was used to join copper piping found in houses built between the 1950s and 1980s. The PVC pipes which initially replaced lead pipes carry their own problems. They can leach toxic chemicals such as vinyl chloride (linked to liver cancer) and organotins (associated with birth defects, damage to the nervous system, and inflammation of the pancreas, memory loss, and insomnia) into the water itself.

Replacing lead pipes with stainless steel or plastic (non-PVC) pipes such as polyethylene is a smart solution. But, if you cannot replace your pipes, the alternative is flushing them of standing water before use, which if done properly could take from two up to five minutes each time.

INSULATING MATERIAL

Asbestos was widely used building material (especially insulating material) due to its heat-resistant properties and was a popular component of a variety of home building and consumer products including vinyl flooring, subflooring, roofing tiles, siding, appliances, such as dryers and stoves, and even ironing board covers and oven mitts, well into the 1970s. It has now become notorious due to its recognized connection to mesothelioma (a chest cancer) and other cancers that afflict the lungs, esophagus, stomach, colon, and pancreas. The disease asbestosis, the buildup of benign scar tissue in the lungs, is also triggered by asbestos.

If you suspect that your home contains asbestos or plan a renovation of a home insulated before the 1970s, always call professional inspectors to collect and analyze samples to determine if they contain asbestos, and never handle materials you suspect contain asbestos!

Fiberglass, cellulose, and cotton are the three types of insulation commonly used today. Fiberglass insulation, in use since the 1930s, accounts for approximately 90 percent of all residential insulation sold and installed in the U.S., according to the North American Insulation Manufacturers Association (NAIMA), and it also accounts for the most substantial and well-documented public health threats of modern insulation. The problem is that poorly installed fiberglass can escape from the insulation, filling the air with the equivalent of microscopic shards of glass. If inhaled, these tiny particles of glass can inflict damage to the lungs. What's more, fiberglass is considered to be a probable carcinogen by the National Institutes of Health. Children are at greater risk than adults when exposed, because they breathe more air (and whatever particles it contains).

Containment is the key to dealing with fiberglass insulation. Removal of existing fiberglass could pose a greater health risk than leaving it in place and sealing it. If properly installed, fiberglass insulation is thought to have little or no health risk. Make sure that fiberglass insulation is not exposed to air-handling ductwork, which would blow microscopic glass particles that make up fiberglass into your breathing space. The fiberglass insulation industry now addresses these concerns by offering encapsulated batts, which seal the fiberglass behind a layer of polyethylene.

FLOORING

Modern flooring is often made of synthetic materials, some of which can emit unhealthy fumes into indoor air. Their adhesives and finishes may compound the problem. These products contain volatile organic compounds (VOCs), which contribute to indoor air pollution. Vinyl flooring is made of polyvinyl chloride (PVC), which may emit the hormone altering and carcinogenic plasticizers known as phthalates, which continually release fumes into the air. This can result in lung disease, and children with PVC flooring in their homes have an 89 percent higher risk of bronchial obstruction than children in PVC-free homes. PVC is also used in wall coverings, countertops, miniblinds, and window frames (as well as many children's toys), and is a toxic substance throughout its life cycle. The manufacture and incineration of PVC create dioxins, known human carcinogens also linked to reproductive and immune disorders. Indeed, exposure to a single PVC fire can cause permanent lung damage. Glues used to fix vinyl flooring may contain nerve-damaging and cancer-triggering solvents such as toluene and benzene.

Fortunately, there are many safe alternatives to synthetic and treated flooring. The first rule is to choose natural and untreated materials. These include natural or "true" linoleum, *untreated* hardwood, cork, ceramic tile, marble, stone slate, and concrete (which can be stained in a variety of colors). For a nursery, resilient flooring (such as true linoleum or cork) is a good alternative to carpeting, absorbing much of the shock of a tumbling baby.

Furniture

Furniture makes our homes comfortable, livable spaces. But whether we're talking about the sofa or a baby's crib, there are a few things to consider about materials used to construct furniture. Both wood and upholstered furniture can contain unhealthy glues, which are used in particleboard, chipboard, pressed wood, and plywood. All of these can emit formaldehyde (a solvent which causes cancer, memory loss, reduced lung function, immune system damage, nausea, and insomnia) and other VOCs for years. Wood furniture finishes, particularly those that are oil-based, may also emit chemicals. Upholstered furniture typically contains polyurethane foam, which may diffuse VOCs as well. This foam and covering fabrics are often treated with chemical-laden finishes for stain resistance, waterproofing, and flame retardancy.

If you've had your furniture for a few years, it's probably already emitted most of its VOCs. When you are considering new furniture, though, you should pay attention to the materials that it's constructed with. Stick to untreated, natural woods. The most deceiving furniture looks like natural wood, but internal pieces, such as drawers, backs, and bottoms may be made of particleboard or plywood. Natural veneers are sometimes used on cheaper, manufactured wood products. Inspect carefully. Unfinished edges are particularly telling.

For upholstered chairs and couches, you can have sofas, love seats, and chairs custom-made with organic cotton and wool fill. Wool is flame retardant and substitutes well for foam used for that purpose. Seeking used furniture, which has already emitted any unhealthy fumes, provides a welcome excuse to go antique hunting. Old upholstered furniture may have accumulated dust. Using a HEPA vacuum cleaner and/or steam cleaning will help get rid of embedded dust.

Since CCA (copper, chromium, and arsenic) treated woods can have a green tint, avoid buying play equipment or outside furniture, such as chairs and decking with a green tint. Naturally hard woods can be used instead of softer woods that are treated with chemicals to make them more durable. And natural oils, such as linseed oil, can be highly effective in preventing damage from pests.

WOOD

Conventional plywood is made of thin veneers of wood that are bonded together with formaldehyde resins. The majority of hardwood plywood, used indoors for cabinetry and paneling, are composed of a core layer faced with higher quality woods using urea-formaldehyde (UF) glue. Softwood plywood is used for exterior and structural applications (walls, floors, roofs), and its adhesive consists of phenol formaldehyde (PF) resin. PF is a more expensive, water-resistant glue, and off-gasses formaldehyde at a relatively slower rate than UF glues. Particleboard, used primarily indoors for furniture and cabinets, is made from wood chips and other plant fibers bonded with formaldehyde-based resins. So it seems that the worst "wood glues" are used inside the home where they do the most harm.

Another problem from wood products is from "pressure treated" or "salt treated" woods. Most wood for use outdoors, in decks, raised beds, and playground equipment, is treated with a combination of chromium, copper, and highly toxic arsenic, or CCA, to preserve it from the elements, insects, and fungi. CCA can migrate to the surface of the wood right after it's applied, forming a white crystalline residue that can be absorbed through the skin. And even though there is a warning label on CCA-treated wood to not use it where food will be prepared, this wood is sometimes used for picnic tables.

Protect your children from the hazards of pressure-treated CCA wood in public parks and playgrounds. Wipe feet on a doormat before going indoors from the deck, and wash children's hands after they spend time on the deck or in the playground. Seal any existing wooden surface treated with chromate copper arsenate (CCA) with paint or a polyurethane coating to trap in arsenic emissions. Repaint every six months, as these coatings don't trap arsenic for more than six months. Do not burn wood treated with CCA as it will release the arsenic as smoke. Do not use it as compost or use it near edible plants. Treat it as hazardous waste and contact your local sanitation department for information on how to dispose of it.

Outside utility poles, fences, and some play equipment can also contain the wood preservatives pentachlorophenol (penta or PCP) and creosote as well as arsenic. These substances are ranked among the most potent cancer agents, promoters of birth defects and reproductive problems, and nervous system toxicants. They contain chemicals that in other contexts are labeled hazardous waste because of the contaminants that are found in them. On a warm day you can really smell these toxic substances because they will evaporate into the air more quickly.

One of the most common forms of wood treatment is used to prevent insect infestation and dry or wet rot. Large amounts of pesticides, such as organophosphates and carbamates and other potentially health damaging and toxic chemicals, are used for this purpose. Many years ago the now banned cancer-causing organochlorine known as Lindane was commonly used as a wood preserver and is still present in many older timbers. Although virtually all of these threats can be minimized or totally prevented via chemical-free methods, such as lowering levels of humidity in the home to discourage the growth of fungi such as dry and wet rot (which flourish in the damp), most people, without thinking, regularly turn to chemicals. Try to deal with dry or wet rot by preventing water from getting through

Chemical-Free Home Renovations

➤ Avoid building products that use adhesives (particularly those with epoxy), paints, or varnishs which emit VOCs. Find the low- or no-VOC alternatives.

➤ If you have to use glue, silicon rubber glue, latex, hide glue, and water washable wood glue are less toxic than epoxy adhesives.

➤ Use sealants made with pure silicone or linseed-oil putty.

➤ Use wooden window frames rather than PVC fittings.

➤ Avoid products that are made of plastics and treated with fire retardants.

➤ If asbestos insulation materials appear soft, crumbly, or otherwise damaged, asbestos may be exposed. Do not touch it. Instead, contact a professional asbestos inspector to collect and analyze samples for asbestos. Do-it-yourselfers should not attempt asbestos repair or removal.

➤ Install a HEPA filter in the bedroom and main living rooms in your home, particularly if it has recently been renovated using modern, chemically treated products.

➤ When building with wood, use solid, untreated hardwood rather than chemically treated softwood such as pine. Also avoid using plywood, MDF (medium density fiberboard), or chipboard.

➤ Seal wood on your deck or home playground equipment containing CCA with paint or a polyurethane coating to trap in arsenic emissions. Be sure your family members wipe their feet and wash their hands after spending time on the deck or a playground with CCA wood.

Did You Know?

➤   Chemical wood preservatives account for the single largest pesticide use in the United States. More than 1.6 billion pounds of wood preservatives were used in 1995, making it the most used pesticide in the United States.

➤   New pressed woods and particleboard products may emit fumes from glues that contain formaldehyde, a suspected carcinogen.

in the first place rather than using chemical treatments. Likewise, find out natural ways of making timber inhospitable to bugs and insects.

Your Garden and Garage

Your shed, garage, or anywhere that you store building and gardening materials, can be a huge source of chemicals. Old cans of paint and varnish are highly volatile and may contain a large number of synthetic chemicals such as plastics, lead, mercury, styrene, and solvents. The good news is that safer alternatives for paints and varnishes that are free from toxic metals and pthalates and contain low levels of VOCs, are now readily available from many environmentally friendly building product retailers.

Cars are a major source of chemicals not only from the burning up of fuel, but from the vast numbers of chemicals used in car maintenance. These include:

➤   Fuel additives (such as numerous extremely noxious substances for cleaning the inside of a car engine) containing pesticides such as organophosphates.

➤   Octane boosters (to prevent knocking) containing lead or manganese.

- ➤ Cooling system additives (mainly used to stop coolant leaks).
- ➤ Oil additives (to reduce friction, prevent burning, prevent leaking, etc.).
- ➤ Engine treatments to prevent friction, containing Teflon and the heavy metal molybdenum.
- ➤ Specialty lubricants, including specialty greases and synthetic lubricants, dielectric grease, silicone-based brake greases, heavy metal–based "moly" greases for lubricating shoepads, and synthetic motor oils. All the above chemicals and additives used in cars should be stored in a well-ventilated (to the outside air), cool place, preferably in sealed containers. Gloves should be used when these substances are handled, or, if this is not practicable, then hands should be washed shortly afterward. Those working with these substances regularly need proper protective clothing, which needs to be left at work or removed before being brought into the home.

Other products found in garages include toxic glues and adhesives that off-gas a range of harmful solvents, as well as phthalates, plastics, and other chlorinated compounds. Natural glues made from animal products are available, which people have been using to glue things together for thousands of years, but are less powerful. Wood preservatives for garden fences and furniture also act as a major source of toxic chemicals.

Your garden is another major source of chemicals in your home environment. To understand how, take a look round any regular garden center and see how many products there are containing poisonous or hazardous substances labels.

A startling 67 million pounds of pesticides are used each year on lawns. Indeed, suburban lawns and gardens receive far heavier pesticide applications per acre than most other land areas in the U.S., including agricultural acres. The problem is that a child in a household that uses home and garden pesticides has a 6.5-percent higher risk of developing leukemia. Dog owners who use the herbicide 2, 4-D four or more times per season double their dog's chances of suffering lymphoma. And of the thirty-six most commonly used lawn pesticides,

A Chemical-Free Garden and Garage

➤   Dispose of any herbicides, weed killers, insect sprays,
    and other noxious substances (responsibly of course),
    and replace them with more environmentally friendly
    products.

➤   To create more natural predators for the insects in your
    garden, leave a pile of logs in your garden so they can hi-
    bernate over winter. You can also create a small area of
    wilderness in your garden that does not get cut, treated
    with chemicals, or cultivated.

➤   Plant a fern near utility poles or any other area near wood
    treated with pressurized CCA, as ferns absorb arsenic.

➤   Talk to a clerk at your local gardening or hardware store
    about chemical-free gardening products and methods.

fourteen are probable or possible carcinogens, fifteen are linked with
birth defects, twenty-one with reproductive effects, twenty-four with
neurotoxicity, and twenty-two with liver or kidney damage.

In addition to the damage done from deliberately applied chemicals,
soil and plants are contaminated by chemicals from pressure–treated
CCA wood in decking, garden furniture, and fencing. Wood treated
with substances such as creosote also emits toxic substances that can
be breathed in.

Fortunately, most of these toxins can be avoided, as evidenced by the
fact that agriculture played such a vital role long before chemicals were
invented. There is already a mountain of information on traditional
horticulture practices from the past. Much of it has been ignored for
years, but a growing number of farmers are reviving older methods to
farm their land and raise their animals organically. If you take your
gardening seriously, there are now lots of books available on organic

horticultural techniques. Another good source of information can be found at the Web site www.organicgardening.com.

Beauty Products

Although you may not realize it, many beauty and personal cleansing products are far from natural. In fact, most are stuffed with synthetic chemicals such as pesticides, preservatives, plastics, fluoride, and artificial scents to make the products smell nicer, feel and look better, and last longer. However, together they all add up to a massive load of poisonous chemicals, the vast majority of which we could all live quite happily without.

Cosmetics

For a long time, people have turned a blind eye when it came to toxic chemicals in cosmetics, added in the name of beauty. Ancient Egyptians used lead and mercury to produce fashionable face-whitening effects, and the practice continued with the early Greek and Roman civilizations. Elizabethan court ladies used arsenic face powder to whiten the skin. These powders, if used excessively, were potentially deadly. But before you scoff at their use of these known, highly dangerous substances, beware that the practice of using toxic substances in cosmetics appears to be still going strong today.

Most consumers would be surprised to learn that the government

Did You Know?

The National Institute of Occupational Safety and Health has found more than 2,500 chemicals in cosmetics that are toxic and that can cause skin and eye irritations, tumors, reproductive complaints, and biological mutations in animals and, therefore, possibly humans.

does not require health studies or premarket testing for cosmetics and other personal care products before they are sold. According to the government agency that regulates cosmetics, the FDA's Office of Cosmetics and Colors, a cosmetics manufacturer may use almost any raw material as a cosmetic ingredient and market the product without an approval from the FDA. The toxicity of product ingredients is scrutinized almost exclusively by a self-policing industry-safety committee known as the Cosmetic Ingredient Review (CIR) panel. Because testing is voluntary and controlled by the manufacturers, many ingredients in cosmetics products are not safety tested at all.

A study by the U.S.-based Environmental Working Group showed that 89 percent of the 10,500 ingredients used in personal-care products have not been evaluated for safety by the CIR, the FDA, or any other publicly accountable institution. The absence of government oversight for this $35 billion industry leads to companies routinely marketing products with ingredients that are poorly studied, not studied at all, or worse, known to pose potentially serious health risks.

Products such as fragrances are not regulated at all. Under the guise of "proprietary information," manufacturers can put anything they want into a fragrance without telling anyone, including the government. So at present, cosmetics are being marketed in the United States containing substances that may pose a serious health hazard.

During our daily personal-care regimen, most of us have exposed ourselves to more than two hundred different chemicals. A recent surge of media attention reveals new concerns about detrimental ingredients that are affecting more than our physical health. An article in a recent

Did You Know?

The FDA cannot require companies to do safety testing of their cosmetic products before marketing.

—*FDA Office of Cosmetics and Colors (FDA 1995)*

USA Weekend reported: "The Environmental Protection Agency (EPA) is increasing research of synthetic chemicals (pesticides, plastics, and industrial mutants) that may be juggling your hormone signals. After reviewing nearly 300 studies, the EPA concluded that ingredients in shampoos, dyes, and other everyday products may be playing havoc with hormones that control reproduction and development."

Chemicals from cosmetics enter our bodies in a number of ways. Powders are the least absorbed through our skin, while oily solutions or those designed to increase moisture allow more of the chemical to be absorbed. Eye makeup can be absorbed by the highly sensitive mucous membranes covering the eyeball. Hair sprays, perfumes, and dusting powders can be inhaled, irritating the lungs. Lipstick is often chewed or licked off and swallowed.

When trying to assess which products are safe and which are dubious, the usually extensive list of ingredients can make things very confusing. However, following their in-depth analysis of the problem, the Environmental Working Group (EWG) has produced a very useful Web site named Skin Deep that provides a safety assessment of ingredients in personal-care products (www.ewg.org/reports/skindeep/browse_products.php). Here you can type in the brand name of your deodorant, toothpaste, soap, shampoo, and whatever else you may use and the site will tell you how many ingredients the products collectively contain and a calculator will rate the aggregate health threat those ingredients may pose to you. Each product is ranked according to its ingredients' potential to:

➤ Cause cancer.
➤ Trigger allergic reactions.
➤ Interfere with the endocrine (hormonal) system.
➤ Impair reproduction or damage a developing fetus.

The existence of any harmful impurities in the product, unstudied ingredients, "penetration enhancers" that help chemicals get absorbed through the skin, or, any violation of industry safety recommendations surrounding its use are also considered when measuring a product's safety.

Read the Label: Dangerous Chemicals
Found in Common Beauty Products

CHEMICAL	COSMETIC	HEALTH RISK
Crystalline Silica	Talcum powder	Known human carcinogen
Coal tar	Shampoos designed to control itching and eczema	Known human carcinogen
Benzyl violet 4B (also known as violet 2)	In more than twenty-five products including shampoos, nail treatments, and moisturizing body bars	Carcinogen
Formaldehyde	In twenty-three products, including menopause creams, hair-thinning serum, antidandruff shampoos, and sun screens	Probable human carcinogen linked to breast cancer and abnormal growth of reproductive tissues
Lead acetate	Hair dye	Known carcinogen and can cause brain damage
Selenium sulfide	Dandruff shampoo	Carcinogen

(continued)

Read the Label: Dangerous Chemicals
Found in Common Beauty Products

CHEMICAL	COSMETIC	HEALTH RISK
Phthalates	Skin moisturizers, nail polish	Causes birth defects in male children
Parabens	Preservatives in blush, mascara, lipstick, hair dye, powder, foundation, concealer, moisturizers, and sunscreen	Can cause breast cancer and birth abnormalities
Sodium lauryl sulfate	Shampoo, body wash, bubble bath, and toothpaste	Contains carcinogenic contaminants, increases the absorption of toxic chemicals
Butylene glycol	Hairspray	Skin irritant
Zirconium	Nail polish	Causes respiratory problems
Potassium bromate	Toothpaste	Causes bleeding and inflammation of gums
Nickel sulfate	Hair dye, astringent	Skin irritant
Resorcinol	Dandruff shampoo	Skin irritant

Choose products made by companies that sell natural, environmentally friendly, or, best of all, organic products, such as Dr. Hauschka. The direct marketing American company known as Shaklee also offers a great range of high-quality natural products. It might take you a little time, effort, and money to find alternatives for your favorite products, but believe me, the rewards will most definitely be worth it.

TOOTHPASTE

Toothpaste can contain a number of harmful ingredients, such as ammonia, benzyl alcohol/sodium benzoate, ethanol, artificial colors and flavors, flouride, formaldehyde, mineral oil, plastic (PVP), and saccharin. Formaldehyde, mineral oil, PVP, and saccharin are all classified as carcinogens or suspected carcinogens, as is flouride, which has been banned in many European countries and is the subject of concern with regard to thyroid problems.

Indeed, studies in recent years have shown that fluoride does *not* reduce cavities, and now scientists are linking fluoride to dental deformity and crippling bone disease. A recent report by the Greater Boston Physicians for Social Responsibility reviews studies showing that fluoride interferes with brain function in young animals and in children, reducing IQ. Some evidence suggests that fluoride causes bone cancer in male rats and perhaps in young men. Some European countries have recently banned most forms of fluoride products and are investigating bans on fluoride toothpaste. In fact, as of April 1997, toothpaste has been required to carry poison control information on the label as even a small amount, like a half a toothpaste tube full, can harm or kill a small child. Fluoride is also a hormone disrupter. Concentrations of fluoride are thought to be high enough in some toothpastes and mouthwashes to promote gingivitis (gum inflammation) as well as oral cancer.

Mouthwash may also contain formaldehyde (a substance that is used to preserve dead bodies) and ammonia. Exposure to ammonia fumes over a long period of time may cause damage to the eyes, liver, kidneys, and lungs, and may cause bronchitis, along with cough, phlegm, and shortness of breath.

An increasing number of companies are beginning to sell fluoride-

Did You Know?

➤ "Hypoallergenic" does not guarantee an absence of allergic reactions, it only minimizes the occurrence of well-known allergens.

➤ "Unscented" does not mean a product contains no fragrance. Ingredients used to mask unpleasant chemical odors do not have to be identified on product labels.

free toothpaste. Most are not yet available in supermarkets though, so check your health food store. I recommend aloe vera/tea tree mint flavor toothpaste made by the company Kingfisher.

DEODORANT

The use of antiperspirant deodorant formulas has been subject to a lot of controversy due to the aluminum base and parabens (chemicals used as preservatives)—among other harsh and toxic substances such as solvents and some fragrances—that are used in many commercial products. Aluminum compounds—particularly aluminum chlorohydrate—are easily absorbed through the skin and have, in the only reported trial to date, already been linked with higher risks of Alzheimer's.

Scientists have now also linked the use of deodorants, particularly antiperspirants, with breast cancer risk in women as they believe parabens could be responsible for accelerating the growth of tumors in the breast. This finding has been strengthened by the fact that a woman is now eight times more likely to develop breast cancer in the area of the breast closest to the underarm than in any other part of the breast tissue. Decades ago, before the widespread use of these substances, breast cancer rates were not only considerably lower, but the cancers appeared more regularly in areas throughout the breast.

During the last few years, numerous health-conscious companies have created products that work well to deodorize sweat, even if they don't prevent perspiration. Using these, combined with good general hygiene, should provide you with more than adequate protection and should alleviate any worries you may have about the safety of standard deodorizing and antiperspiration products.

Tom's of Maine makes a great natural deodorant, which is also amazingly free of aluminum and the load of other unwanted nasties normally found in deodorants. I prefer their unscented Nature's Deodorant (you may initially catch a mild whiff of coriander when first putting it on), which has the rare characteristics of being both highly effective and safe. But, naturally scented versions of these are also available. Be cautious of "natural" deodorant crystals as they may contain aluminum, and would therefore not be something you would want to use. Most good health food stores, like my local one, Sunseeds, in Cocoa Beach, Florida, are very helpful and can get most things in for you if they don't already have them in stock.

MEDICATED SHAMPOOS

Medicated shampoos specifically designed for head infestations such as nits and lice may contain powerful insecticides, which when put directly onto the skin are absorbed straight into our bodies. Alternative methods such as fine-tooth combing and natural remedies are not only more effective (as increasing numbers of these parasites have now developed a resistance to many chemicals), but are totally safe.

Regular shampoos as well as antidandruff shampoos can also contain the possible carcinogen formaldehyde as a preservative, listed on the label as "quaternium-15." Formaldehyde is also known to induce asthma attacks, skin rashes, and headaches. Dandruff shampoos may also contain coal tar, although in some cases it seems that this known cancer-causing ingredient is not always revealed on the label. Some dandruff shampoos may also contain resorcinol, a chemical that is easily absorbed through the skin and scalp and that can lead to inflammation of the inner eyelids, irritation of the skin, dizziness, rapid heartbeats, breathing difficulties, unconsciousness, and convulsions.

Many mainstream dandruff shampoos, even if they are free from coal tar, contain other potentially hazardous ingredients such as sodium laureth sulfate or polyethylene glycol (PEG) compounds, both of which are frequently contaminated with a clear-cut carcinogen, 1,4-dioxane. Some even contain cocamide DEA, another suspected carcinogen. Other common agents used to treat dandruff include ketoconazole (an antifungal drug), zinc pyrithione (a toxic substance), and selenium sulfide (a carcinogen).

Luckily, there is a completely safe alternative. Dandruff occurs when the scalp sheds larger than normal amounts of dead epidermal cells. For many years dandruff has been associated with the presence of yeast/fungi of the genus *Malassezia* or *Pityrosporum*. Effective therapy of dandruff has been linked to agents that inhibit these organisms.

ANTI-BACTERIAL PRODUCTS

Antibacterial soap and hand wash commonly contain the antibacterial product known as triclosan, as do many cleansers for preventing acne (acne is thought to be caused by certain bacteria). However, not only does triclosan kill bacteria, it also has been shown to kill human cells.

Antibacterial ingredients have become so prevalent in the United States that there are now antibacterial soaps, personal care preparations, laundry detergents, shampoos, toothpastes, body washes, dish soaps,

Beware of Preservatives

Preservatives in cosmetics extend shelf life by preventing bacterial contamination. Formaldehyde, methyl, and propyl paraben are used in a wide range of traditional cosmetics. Avoid all products containing these preservatives and opt for those that use natural alternatives such as antioxidants like vitamin E. Because natural preservatives only last for six months to one year, you should refrigerate products like natural creams and lotions. Some natural-beauty-product companies embed high gauss magnets into product jars that create magnetic fields that are hostile to bacteria.

and many household cleaning products. The first major test done in people's homes found that using antibacterial products apparently offers little protection against the most common germs. In the study, published in March 2004 in the journal *Annals of Internal Medicine,* it was found that people who used antibacterial soaps and cleansers developed a cough, runny nose, sore throat, fever, vomiting, diarrhea, and other symptoms such as acne, just as often as people who used products that did not contain antibacterial ingredients. What's more, many traditional medical circles now accept the hygiene hypothesis that states that children need to be exposed to some bacteria in early childhood in order to strengthen their immune systems. Children who are not exposed to common bacteria, which are wiped out by antibacterial soap, may be more prone to allergies and asthma. All you actually need to use to remove bacteria safely is a plain, chemical-free soap that you can pick up in your local health food store.

SUNSCREEN

Octyomethoxycinnamate (OMC) is an important ingredient in 90 percent of the world's sunscreen lotions. Alarmingly, this chemical has been shown to actually kill living cells. Titanium dioxide, a compound whose toxicity remains unclear, is another ingredient found in many sunscreens. Researchers now say the chemical can be absorbed by human skin. Titanium dioxide is a fine, white powder used in sunscreens because of its ability to reflect and scatter ultraviolet light. The compound's full effects on human health are still under investigation. The U.S. government's National Institute for Occupational Safety and Health (NIOSH) labels the chemical "a potential occupational carcinogen."

While we all actually need to get out in the sun to produce vitamin D and remain healthy, we don't need too much at one time as this can be harmful. Indeed while sunscreen does appear to prevent sunburn, it does not seem to prevent the skin cancer known as melanoma. Due to the fact that it encourages people to stay out longer in the sun, it might even increase the risk of melanoma. The best way forward is to limit sun exposure until your system adjusts by increasing melanin pigmentation in the skin. Also, taking antioxidants increases skin protection against sun-induced radiation damage. So avoid sunscreens or minimize their use, as they could in themselves increase your risk of disease.

AFTERSHAVE

Aftershave is notorious for containing a host of chemicals that can be harmful to your skin, the very thing it is advertised to protect. There are also many substances in aftershave that can cause a host of other illnesses and diseases. When buying an aftershave product, be sure to avoid the following:

➤ **Benzyl acetate:** Linked to pancreatic cancer and may be absorbed through the skin.
➤ **Ethyl acetate:** May cause damage to the liver and kidneys, headaches, and dehydration of the skin.
➤ **Terpineol:** May cause pneumonitis or even fatal edema if breathed into the lungs, central-nervous-system and respiratory damage, and headaches.

Similarly, shaving foams and creams may contain harmful substances such as:

➤ **Benzaldehyde:** A central-nervous-system suppressant that may cause skin, eye, and lung irritation, nausea, abdominal pain, and kidney damage.
➤ **Camphor:** Can cause irritation of the eyes, nose, and throat, nausea, and even convulsions if inhaled or rubbed on the skin.
➤ **Ethanol:** Can cause irritation to the upper respiratory tract, even in low concentrations, as well as central-nervous-system disorder if inhaled or ingested.
➤ **Limonene:** Carcinogenic; must not be inhaled.
➤ **Linalool:** Has been linked to respiratory disturbances. Animal studies have also linked it to reduced spontaneous motor activity and depressed heart activity.
➤ **g-Terpinene:** Can provoke asthmatic attacks.

Did You Know?

➤ Bubble bath soaps (bath foam) almost always contain sodium lauryl sulfate (which can be contaminated with carcinogens from chemical processing), formaldehyde (possibly cancer causing), and many chemical perfumes.

➤ Lipsticks contain petroleum distillates, which can cause damage to the nervous system, skin, kidneys, and eyes. They also contain aluminum, a known toxin.

➤ Talcum powder was linked in a 1982 article in the journal *Cancer* to a 328 percent increased risk of ovarian cancer for women who apply it to sanitary napkins and genitals.

➤ Hair dyes, both permanent and temporary, often contain a host of toxic chemicals, with the most toxic ones tending to being found in the darker colored dyes.

PART II

The Chemical Connection to Chronic Illness

CHAPTER 5

Immune System Diseases

THE BODY'S NATURAL DEFENSE SYSTEM, commonly referred to as the immune system, is one of the most important systems we have for protecting our health. Unfortunately, previously rare immune system diseases such as asthma, a relatively unheard of disease at the beginning of the twentieth century, now affect between 100 and 150 million people worldwide. The number of deaths caused by asthma in America has doubled since the early 1980s. Far from stabilizing, it is clear that the situation is in free-fall.

Changes in the immune system, like those that result in asthma, have occurred far too rapidly to have arisen solely as a result of changes in our genetic makeup. It is far more likely that changes in the environment and our diet are at the heart of the new immune system vulnerabilities and disease.

Extensive research now shows that the majority of the most common types of chemicals we are exposed to on a daily basis damage virtually every aspect of our immune system. Indeed there is now a separate branch of medicine, known as immunotoxicology, which specializes in this field alone.

In this chapter, you will learn about the way in which chemicals cause either an underactive or overactive immune system or sometimes both at the same time. The resulting immune system imbalances can have a triggering or exacerbating effect on illnesses such as the common cold and flu, allergies, asthma, hayfever, autoimmune disease, and eczema. The good news is that by following the Toxic Overload program you can start halting these diseases in their tracks and start repairing any existing chemically induced damage previously inflicted on your immune system.

Pesticides, toxic metals, environmental pollutants, solvents, and other chemicals possess powerful immune system–destroying qualities. They appear to damage the smooth functioning of the immune system in two main ways: suppressing it (immunosuppression) and causing it to be underactive, or sending it into overdrive so that it is overactive.

Common Diseases Associated with a Malfunctioning Immune System

Allergies

Arthritis

Asthma

Autoimmune disorders

Cancer

Connective tissue disorders

Diabetes

Eczema

Food allergies

Hayfever

Infections

Inflammatory disorders

Urticaria, or hives

If suppressed, the immune system cannot work properly to fight invading bodies—the immune system's primary responsibility—and as a result, the body becomes more vulnerable to infections and is at greater risk of developing not just colds, flus, and common illnesses, but also more serious diseases like cancer. Immune system overdrive causes a different set of problems including a host of allergic reactions, such as hives, runny nose, wheezing, and in extreme cases anaphylactic shock. It also increases the long-term chances of developing any of the autoimmune system disorders (see page 128). Below you will find a description of how chemicals have an impact on a wide range of illnesses and conditions including allergies, asthma, autoimmune disease, hayfever, and more.

Immunosuppresion: Not Just Colds and Flus

Your doctor will probably be able to name quite a few nonchemical factors such as stress, surgery, and certain infections that are known to suppress the immune system. However, the significant role chemicals play in suppressing the immune system is often overlooked by the medical community. This is a major problem in light of the recent World Resources Institute (WRI) report that came to the staggering conclusion that pesticides are a likely cause of immune suppression for millions of people throughout the world.

This is of great relevance because we are all exposed to these immune system–suppressing pesticides at every turn, in everything from the food we eat to the fly spray we use around the house. However, it is not just the pesticides that we currently use that cause these problems—some of the worst offenders are chemicals that were banned decades ago but persist in our environment and can still be found in our foods.

A classic example of this is the group of chemicals known as organochlorines, which were previously designed as pesticides but are now a widespread environmental pollutant. Because these chemicals tend to be absorbed into living plants and animals, predators such as trout and salmon tend to contain particularly high levels of them.

To illustrate the extent to which polluted foods can cause real damage to our immune systems, we need to turn to a study that took place in a remote part of the Canadian Arctic. Despite being an undeveloped, nonindustrialized area, researchers found that the local women and their offspring had relatively high levels of organochlorines, heavy metals, and other toxic chemicals in their bodies, which was found to be due to the large proportion of seafood in their diet. The higher the levels of pollutants the babies were exposed to in the womb, the higher the incidence of ear infections they would get as infants, illustrating the resistance-lowering capacity of these chemicals.

There are many other drugs which suppress the immune system—indeed, certain chemical compounds are so good at causing immuno-

Chemical Subtances Known to Cause Immunosuppression

Cancer treatments: e.g., chemotherapy

Drugs: steroids, antimalarials, certain antibiotics, certain HIV drugs (e.g., AZT), recreational drugs, azathioprine and cyclosporin, immunosuppressive drugs, and nonsteroidal anti-inflammatory drugs (NSAIDs)

Environmental pollutants: PCBs, dioxin, and endocrine disruptors

Fluoride and chlorine

Infections: malaria, HIV, and salmonella

Pesticides: particularly organochlorines and organophosphates

Solvents

Toxic metals: mercury, as in many vaccinations and amalgam dental fillings, nickel, lead, cadmium, and organotin

suppression, they are used in medicine for these very qualities. For example, steroids possess such powerful immunosuppressive actions that they are deliberately used in organ transplant patients to prevent tissue rejection. Problems arise when steroids are used to treat other conditions, such as cancer, due to the accompanying suppression of the immune system, which can increase the risk of life-threatening infections.

Allergies:
An Overactive Immune System

If contact with certain substances makes your skin red, inflamed, and lumpy, or rapidly affects your ability to breathe, you are not alone. Chances are that you are one among a huge population of people who suffer from health problems and allergies caused by an overactive immune system. Allergic reactions can range from hives to angioedema (swelling beneath the skin) to anaphylactic shock (a severe and rapid allergic systemic reaction following contact with an allergen). With allergic difficulties being potentially fatal, having an overactive immune system can prove just as serious a problem as having an underactive one.

Due to the rapid appearance of allergy symptoms following contact with a particular substance, most people who suffer allergic reactions have a good idea of the substances or factors that make their body react in this dramatic and often alarming way. Most doctors concentrate on common allergens such as foods (especially nuts), pollens, grasses, dust, and bee stings, and instruct patients on how to avoid their allergy triggers. But many doctors fail to recognize the underlying change in our immune systems that has occurred over the years due to chemical poisoning, and that has made us increasingly susceptible to these allergens. These changes not only have raised our chances of becoming "allergic" in the first place, but they increase the number and severity of attacks.

For instance, chemicals like the toxic metals, with mercury and aluminum being prime examples, cause our immune systems to overreact by artificially activating the immune system cells designed to fight intruders

Vaccines: Using Toxic Metals to Stimulate the Immune System

Not only can chemicals act to trigger hives, angioedema, and anaphylactic reaction, but daily exposure to these substances can also cause marked, long-term immune system damage, increasing the chances of developing allergies in the first place. Indeed they are so good at causing the immune system to go into overdrive that some chemicals are actually used for this same purpose in vaccines.

For over sixty years, chemicals have been deliberately added to vaccines to boost the immune response to the bug or pathogen (such as tetanus or flu) that is used in the vaccine. These chemicals are known as adjuvants. Two of the most common in use are the toxic metals aluminum and mercury. Unfortunately, not only does the addition of the toxic metal boost the response to the desired pathogen, it has the side effect of stimulating many other different mechanisms of the immune system that can exacerbate eczema and inflammatory bowel diseases.

The problem is that children are now expected to receive an ever-increasing number of vaccines, leading to a greater buildup of toxic metals in the body. Over the long term, this results in an overstimulated immune system that is more prone to developing an entire range of allergic disorders. In light of the dozens of vaccines that infants are now subjected to, is it any surprise that more children than ever before are allergy sufferers?

or foreign objects or substances. This effectively puts the immune system in perpetual fighting mode. Another effect of this overstimulation of our defense systems is that it triggers the buildup of substances that the fighting cells use as weapons. As these substances, known as cytokines, have the effect of amplifying any potential fight, a higher level of them results in allergic episodes becoming more severe. So in other

Chemical Substances Known to Trigger an Allergic Reaction and Underlying Immune System Imbalances

Chlorine in drinking water and swimming pools

Cigarette smoke

Drugs, such as aspirin, antibiotics, painkillers, and insect repellents

Environmental pollutants (dioxins and PCBs)

Fluoride in water and dental treatments

Food preservatives, colorings, and other additives

Latex rubber

Pesticides (particularly synthetic pyrethroids, organophosphates, carbamates, and organochlorines)

Plastics

Solvents (such as formaldehyde and xylene)

Sunscreen, perfumes, and other toiletry components

Surgical prosthetic implants

Toxic metals (e.g., mercury and aluminum)

Wood preservatives

words, chemicals appear to turn our immune cells into bullies, giving them the weapons and the drive to actually go out and look for a fight.

Chemicals also can increase the chances of developing new allergies. This is because they directly reduce the immune system's ability to differentiate between foreign substances that pose a real threat and those with much lesser toxicities that it may have tolerated for years. So when exposure to immune-damaging chemicals reaches a certain level, the immune system is sent into fight mode. This overreaction throws it off balance and the body starts objecting to substances it has previously tolerated, like foods—resulting in new food allergies—or its very own tissues—resulting in autoimmune diseases. The degree to which your immune system is damaged by chemicals is not only directly related to your level of contamination, but also to your genetic makeup and nutritional status, as suboptimal levels of nutrients (such as magnesium and zinc) can make the immune system more reactive and hyperactive. In fact, many nutrients, such as magnesium and vitamin C, can act as natural antihistamines, effectively calming down a revved-up immune system.

Asthma—Reclaiming the Breath of Life

Asthma is a respiratory illness caused by the inflammation of the air passages in the lungs. During attacks, airways swell and narrow, reducing the flow of air into and out of the lungs.

Asthma is becoming one of the most prevalent illnesses affecting twenty-first-century society. The scale of the problem, not only in the United States but worldwide, is simply staggering. The World Health Organization (WHO) has recently estimated that between 100 and 150 million people around the globe suffer from asthma. Even more troubling, this number is rising quickly. In the United States the overall prevalence of asthma increased from 3.1 percent in 1980 to 5.4 percent in 1994, with the incidence among impoverished inner-city children being much higher. The combined prevalence of diagnosed and undiagnosed asthma among inner-city children at nine to twelve years of age has been estimated at 26 percent and 27 percent in Detroit and San Diego, respectively.

The great question is, what is behind this rise in asthma rates? While scientists are struggling to find an answer, the sales of asthma suppressant drugs have never been better. Despite being good at suppressing attacks, these drugs have not been designed to tackle the problem of what makes someone develop asthma in the first place.

Most experts agree that asthma is a multifactorial problem comprised of a mixture of components, including those that are hereditary, allergic, environmental, infectious, emotional, and nutritional, not to mention that it can be triggered by pharmaceutical drugs, cigarette smoke, and exercise. While it is vital to minimize the exposure to the factors that trigger asthma, this is only part of the problem.

The real issue, which has been pretty much ignored till now, is the fact that our increased exposure to modern artificial chemicals, in combination with an increasingly nutrient-deficient diet, appears to be damaging the health of our immune system by making it hypersensitive and overreactive to substances that it could previously tolerate (see page 117). In fact, Dr. Anthony Seaton from the University of Aberdeen in Scotland believes the dramatic recent rise in asthma incidence could be due to a more "toxic" environment and a more susceptible population.

The existence of a more susceptible population also appears to make sense because our diets are becoming ever more highly processed and nutrient deficient. Our bodies are therefore failing to get even the

Chemicals Linked to Asthma

Air pollutants (nitrogen dioxide, ozone, and sulphur dioxide)

Chlorine and fluoride

Drugs (aspirin and nonsteroidal anti-inflammatory drugs)

Food additives (tartrazine, or yellow dye)

Pesticides (organophosphates and carbamates)

Plastics

Solvents (diesel)

Toxic metals (mercury, lead, platinum salts, nickel, chromium, and cobalt)

basic levels of nutrients they need to work properly. The consequence of this is that people are becoming less and less able to neutralize and rid themselves of the increased load of asthma-inducing toxins that they are being exposed to, resulting in more and more people becoming asthmatic.

How Chemicals Trigger Asthma

Increased chemical exposure can be linked to asthma in two ways. First, chemicals upset the underlying immune system, making it over-reactive and hypersensitive to asthma-provoking allergens such as pollen. Second, they can directly trigger an asthma attack by causing the release of an inflammatory substance in the airways.

Toxic metals are some of the most powerful asthma-inducing agents because they damage the underlying immune system, vulnerable to asthma-provoking allergens. Mercury tends to be found in much higher levels in the bodies of those who have asthma. As the body levels of mercury increase with the number of fillings in a person's mouth, it may not be surprising to hear that people participating in a study in which mercury amalgam fillings were removed experienced a great improvement in their asthma symptoms.

Not only do pesticides increase the long-term risk of getting asthma but they can also trigger acute asthma attacks. Studies examining the effects of pesticides on farmers have revealed that organophosphates and carbamates have the most powerful asthma-inducing effects. As these are some of the pesticides most commonly used in food production, when you eat certain foods you may be unknowingly exposing yourself to a small but potent shot of asthma-triggering chemicals.

Air pollution is a well-known factor linked to higher rates of asthma due to the particulate matter containing heavy metals and the higher levels of solvents present from diesel and its exhaust products and ozone. Studies show that the greater the air pollution, the higher the level of hospital admissions for asthma.

The commonly used water disinfectant chlorine is another chemical commonly linked to asthma. To get an indication of how toxic it is to our lungs, you only have to go back to the reason why it was used as a weaponized gas in the First World War—a powerful lung irritant, it disabled people by targeting their lungs. This is why people who work around and swim regularly in pools that use chlorine as a water disinfectant are thought to be more prone to developing asthma.

Due to the powerful role that chemicals play in triggering asthma, it is a good idea to generally reduce your overall exposure to these toxins (see chapter 3). In addition to eating cleaner foods that are less processed and less polluted and filtering your water, eating foods high in soluble fiber will help lower the existing body burden of asthma-inducing toxins.

Hayfever

Hayfever, otherwise known as allergic rhinitis, is now one of the most common non–life threatening health problems. It affects more than 20 percent of individuals in all age groups worldwide and 25 percent of the U.S. population. Not only does it drive you mad, but it has serious drawbacks for society due to higher health-care expenditure as well as decreased productivity through lost days of school or work. Some people suffer not only in spring and summer, but all year round.

As with asthma, the incidence of hayfever has been steadily rising over the last few decades. While sales of powerful suppressive medications are booming and look set to increase to ever-greater heights, they totally fail to tackle the real cause of the problem. Their benefits are also won at a cost, because the antihistamines, decongestants, anticholinergic agents, and corticosteroid drug therapy typically used in the treatment of allergic rhinitis often have problematic side effects that include sedation, impaired learning/memory, and cardiac arrhythmias. For many, especially children, the health price paid for a dry nose could potentially be unacceptably high.

Hayfever is an allergic condition triggered by various substances, like pollen, synthetic drugs, air pollution, and food sensitivities, leading to sneezing, nasal congestion, constant dripping of the nose, and inflammation of the eyes and sinuses. People tend to suffer from two main forms: the seasonal type, where symptoms occur mainly through-out the height of the pollen season, and the perennial type, which is ex-perienced all year round. Hayfever tends to be a long-term or chronic problem that conventional medicine has no apparent means of pre-venting. Few of the children who develop it will grow out of it. In fact, all modern medicine can do is suppress the symptoms with powerful and often toxic prescription and over-the-counter drugs and suggest people avoid the triggers.

There is increasing evidence that our more polluted environment in combination with a poorer, nutrient-deficient diet is damaging our im-mune systems. The end result seems to be that we are becoming more prone to developing problems such as hayfever. The upshot of this is that our immune system is more susceptible and hyperreactive to aller-gens. Therefore, reducing the overall chemical exposure could not only bring about short-term relief, but longer-term resolution too.

CHEMICAL TRIGGERS OF HAYFEVER

The nose and sinuses are particularly vulnerable to chemical dam-age because they are often the first to be exposed to pollutants and the first to show evidence of chemical damage. The membranes of the nose are also more porous, and therefore they absorb a great amount of pollutants. Consequently, hayfever symptoms are commonly the first sign of chemical sensitivity. In fact, before developing more seri-ous chemical-related diseases, most people have a previous history of hayfever or rhinitis. So if you get a runny nose after breathing in pol-luted air, this is a wonderful opportunity to take seriously and tackle your chemical exposure before your symptoms progress to something more serious.

The types of chemicals linked to hayfever, which are similar to those linked to asthma, can be found on page 125. You don't have to be ex-posed to these chemicals in the air to be affected as they can be found in foods, drinks, and skin-care products, as well as other substances such as dental amalgam and glues. How they enter your body does not impact the damage they can do.

Known Chemical Triggers of Hayfever

Chlorine

Diesel fuel

Newspaper print

Perfumes

Pesticides

Plastics

Solvents

Synthetic drugs

Toxic metals (mercury, lead, nickel, cadmium, chromium)

To limit your exposure to hayfever-inducing chemicals, it is important to take nutritional supplements to help your body lower its existing load of chemicals (vitamin C and magnesium also act as natural antihistamines), and follow the guidelines in chapter 3 when planning and preparing your meals. You should eat organic foods and wash and prepare them in ways that will reduce your chemical intake. Avoid inhaling chemical substances: if you can smell them, they are already in your nose and body.

Eczema: More Than Skin Deep

My first three children have all, at one stage or another, developed eczema. So you can imagine that ever since the first one was diagnosed, I have been at great pains to discover what causes this painful and disfiguring problem, and have sought out all possible ways of treating it.

The more I have discovered about what causes it, the easier it becomes to prevent. The result of my quest is that, to date, all my children are eczema free, without so much as a whiff of steroid cream.

Eczema is now thought to affect an alarming 13 percent of people at some stage during their lives, causing distress and irritation in all those whom it afflicts. By understanding what is causing the spread of this disease, you will realize that there is a positive and effective way forward to tackle eczema, using safe and natural methods.

Eczema, also commonly referred to as dermatitis, is a skin condition characterized by an itchy, red rash. In many cases the skin can become scaly, crack, and weep. The accompanying itchiness is not just annoying, the scratching that frequently accompanies it can increase the chances of infection. In infancy it is commonly found on the face, behind the ears, and on the trunk. In childhood, it tends to settle to the back of the knees and front of the elbows, wrists, and ankles. In adults, the face and the trunk are once more involved. Although many children grow out of it, for many it can remain a long-term or chronic problem.

There are two main types of eczema:

➤ Allergic eczema—when the body develops eczema as a reaction to certain allergens, such as a type of food in the diet.
➤ Irritant contact eczema—when eczema is triggered following direct skin contact with certain irritants such as metals and chemicals.

While conventional medicine has many powerful drugs in its armory to suppress eczema, it has few means of preventing it from occurring in the first place. As a result, ever-greater numbers of people are being subjected to powerful steroid creams that, in addition to having the unwanted side effect of making the skin thinner, can further increase the risk of infection due to their immune-suppressive actions. While these toxic drugs can be very effective at suppressing the symptoms in the short term, if we are to have any chance of finding a long-term cure to this problem, we need to examine why we are becoming more and more vulnerable to this disease in the first place.

CHEMICAL CAUSES OF ECZEMA

At the heart of these abnormal responses appears to lie a damaged immune system. As with all the previously discussed immune disorders, increased levels of chemicals in our bodies in combination with an increasingly nutrient-deficient diet appears to damage the innate balance of the immune system, making it oversensitive to a wide range of eczema-triggering factors both biological and chemical.

Much of the existing work in this field is based on extensive research already done on the large number of people developing eczema as a consequence of handling chemicals as part of their work. Eczema from direct skin contact with chemicals has proved a huge problem because skin can absorb up to 60 percent of a substance such as a cream that is applied to it. With such a potentially large volume of chemicals entering the body through the skin, not only does the total body load increase, making the underlying immune system more vulnerable to diseases such as eczema, but there is plenty of opportunity for these chemicals to trigger a local response on the skin. The inset "Chemicals That Trigger Eczema" shows the types of chemicals that are known to trigger eczema in this way.

Chemicals That Trigger Eczema

Chlorine

Fragrances

Mineral oils

Pesticides

Pharmaceutical drugs

Plastics (resins, rubber chemicals)

Solvents (turpentine)

Toxic metals (mercury, nickel, gold, cobalt, chromate)

It seems likely that early damage to our immune system could be at the very heart of the recent rise in eczema rates. Evidence suggests that exposure of the fetus to higher levels of chemicals in the womb damages the immune system, making it more reactive to eczema-inducing triggers for life. The subsequent increased exposure to toxins throughout life can increase the tendency to develop eczema even further. So it seems that our children can be in effect "programmed" to develop eczema even before they are even born (see Asthma on page 120). With the level of pollution on the increase, it seems that the number of people who will suffer from eczema is likely to get even higher.

Autoimmune Diseases

Our immune system is our body's highly effective defense, designed to kill foreign bodies, such as harmful bacteria. Autoimmune diseases are caused when our immune system fails to differentiate between foreign invaders and the body tissues it has been programmed to protect. This is potentially devastating, as once a particular type of tissue is labeled as an enemy, the immune system will target it for destruction and unleash its full might against it forever. Autoimmune diseases include rheumatoid arthritis, juvenile diabetes, ankylosing spondylitis, systemic lupus erythematosis (lupus or SLE), scleroderma, Hashimoto's thyroiditis, primary myxoedema, thyrotoxicosis, and Addison's disease.

If you have read the beginning of this chapter, you will know by now that we are seeing an increase in all the major diseases of the immune system. Autoimmune diseases are no different as these once-rare diseases are now affecting more and more people. For instance, deaths from previously rare diseases such as lupus rose from 879 to 1,406 over the last twenty years. While heredity plays an important role in passing on autoimmune diseases, an increasing number of people without a genetic link to autoimmune diseases are developing them. Researchers are beginning to discover that exposure to toxic chemicals is playing a major part in this autoimmune system disease epidemic.

The connection between chemicals and autoimmune diseases was first noticed when people who were exposed to larger amounts of certain chemicals because of their jobs, habits, or even medical treatment were found to be at greater risk of developing autoimmune diseases. For example, workers exposed to silica dust have tended to have much higher rates of rheumatoid arthritis, lupus, scleroderma, and glomerulonephritis (inflammation of the kidneys). Silica dust is commonly found in minerals such as quartz, tridymite, and cristobalite, and silica is used in industry as an abrasive cleaner and an inert filler. It can be

Chemicals That Have Been Linked to Autoimmune Diseases

➤ Estrogen replacement therapy in postmenopausal women has been linked to lupus, scleroderma, and Raynaud's disease (sudden decreased blood circulation in fingers or toes).

➤ Oral contraceptives may also play a role in promoting lupus.

➤ Industrial exposure to silica dust increases the risk of scleroderma, rheumatoid arthritis, glomerulonephritis, and lupus.

➤ Solvent exposure has been investigated as a risk factor for scleroderma.

➤ Mercury has been strongly linked to kidney disease, such as glomerulonephritis, multiple sclerosis–like diseases, and chronic polyarthritis.

➤ Hair products and certain medications that contain a similar chemical (aromatic amines) are linked to lupus.

➤ Gold, a common treatment of rheumatoid arthritis, appears to promote autoimmune disorders.

found in scouring powder and metal polish, and is used as an extender in paint, as wood filler, in concrete, and as a component in road-surfacing mixtures.

When this connection was examined more closely, it was discovered that not only can these chemicals trigger a wide range of autoimmune diseases, but they can also exacerbate existing ones. So how is this thought to have come about?

How Chemicals Trigger Autoimmune Diseases

As the chemicalization of our world has resulted in the rise of our overall body burden of toxins, the natural balance of our immune system is becoming increasingly disturbed. Chemical exposure can upset the natural balance of the immune system by increasing the level of immune system activity (see page 117). If chemical exposure continues over the long term, this imbalance causes a new set of problems, the most obvious being tissue inflammation, resulting from a greater level of the tissue dissolving/inflammatory substances known as cytokines that are produced by an activated immune system. The other serious consequence is damage to the mechanisms enabling the immune system to differentiate between friend and foe, and the increased production of autoantibodies. While it is good to produce antibodies, the substance produced by our immune system to attack invading or foreign substances, *auto*antibodies are antibodies programmed to attack our own body tissues.

Autoimmune diseases arise when our body starts acting on these false instructions and tries to kill body tissues that, due to the production of autoantibodies, become falsely labeled as foreign tissues.

Once your body's immune system takes a dislike to a certain part of your body, it will target it for destruction using all the methods at its disposal. Once initiated, this process carries on until it succeeds in killing its target. If it targets a particular organ such as your thyroid gland, as in the case of Hashimoto's thyroiditis, the amount of thyroid hormone your body produces will be severely reduced. Although this causes many difficulties, the presence of thyroid hormone replacements makes it relatively easy to deal with this situation. However, things get much more difficult if the tissues that the autoantibodies attack are more widespread, such as in the case of lupus, when autoantibodies to DNA are created. Since DNA is a protein present in every living cell in the body, the disease symptoms will be much more widespread and difficult to deal with.

While you cannot rid yourself of an autoimmune system disease, it is possible to calm down an overrevved immune system by reducing the levels of toxic chemicals in your body. This can be an effective way of putting the brakes on disease progression and keeping symptoms to a minimum. It will also help lower your chances of developing another autoimmune disease.

Taking the nutritional supplements outlined in the supplement program in chapter 2, you can further fortify your immune system while simultaneously protecting your body from the harmful effects of toxic chemicals. Although it is best to follow the complete program, the nutrients that are particularly important in calming down the immune system are zinc, selenium, magnesium, and vitamins A, B, C, D, and E.

However, I have found that some people with thyroid diseases have problems taking certain supplements, particularly if they are on thyroid hormone replacements. So I would strongly advise you to consult your doctor before embarking on a course of supplements. Or, better still, consult a doctor who specializes in environmental medicine, as he or she will be more used to administering nutritional supplements to people who have health problems and may already be on powerful immune system–suppressing drugs.

Rebalancing the Immune System

The Toxic Overload program will lower the body's exposure to chemical toxins and give the immune system the nutrients it needs to work properly. Best of all, by ridding your home and body of chemicals, you will strengthen the immune system naturally, letting it work the way that nature intended. Not only should this dramatically increase your resistance to infections, but it should also make the immune system less reactive to substances such as pollen or foods and alleviate the distressing symptoms of many autoimmune diseases. Reducing inflammation will also help lower your dependence on drugs, such as steroids, that are commonly used to suppress an overactive immune system.

Whether your aim is to strengthen your immune system to reduce the number of coughs and colds you are getting, control your allergies, or increase your ability to fight cancer, it is vital that you lower your overall exposure to chemicals—whether they are in the form of environmental toxins or medications—that cause imbalance in your immune system.

I am not for one moment suggesting that you stop medical treatment for potentially life-threatening problems, but I am suggesting that you review with your doctor the need for all the drugs you are taking, and only take those thought to be essential for your health. For instance, if you are going on a vacation, choosing a place where you will not have to take immune-suppressing antimalarial drugs will mean you avoid exposing yourself to their immune-depressive actions. The key is to use the information in this book to work with your doctor to prevent unnecessary damage to your immune system.

SUPPLEMENTS

As well as lowering your exposure to toxic chemicals, it is vitally important to ensure that you are getting enough nutrients. If vital nutrient levels fall, the immune system can become suppressed or overactive. And if nutritional deficiency continues for any length of time, it also increases your chance of developing one of the many autoimmune diseases. The supplement program in chapter 2 is perfect for rebalancing your immune system: it will help boost an underperforming immune system and suppress an overactive one.

The main nutrients needed for proper immune function are the vitamins A, B_6, C, D, and E, biotin, and folic acid; the minerals magnesium, zinc, iron, copper, and selenium; the omega-3 and omega-6 fatty acids; and a sufficient and high-quality supply of proteins. Magnesium, zinc, iron, and vitamin A seem to be most critical to proper immune system balance. For example, low levels of the mineral zinc can reduce the ability of certain parts of the immune system to work properly by up to 70 percent. Unfortunately, people in both the developed and developing worlds are most commonly deficient in these nutrients.

But deficiency is not the only risk: slightly lower or suboptimal levels of these nutrients will also reduce the functioning of the immune system. This means that the vast majority of the nonsupplementing population, as well as many who are supplementing, but inadequately, are effectively putting themselves at risk for a weakened immune system. But when nutrients such as amino acids (proteins), omega-3 fatty acids, and vitamins, particularly E, C, and A, are taken in excess of what is simply needed to prevent deficiency, they appear to have remarkable immune-system boosting effects.

At the Department of Surgery, College of Medicine, University of Cincinnati, megadoses of several of the above vitamins and other nutrients were given to patients admitted for surgical procedures. Not only were infectious complications in these surgical patients reduced by approximately 75 percent, but the duration of their hospital stay was reduced by more than 20 percent.

Nutrient supplementation can also help rebalance the immune system and remove chemicals that overstimulate it. The net result of long-term supplementation is fewer immune reactions and reactions that are less severe. Taking nutrients can also help suppress allergy symptoms in the shorter term since many, such as vitamin C and magnesium, act as natural antihistamines.

DIET

To cleanse your body of unwanted toxins and encourage optimum immune function, follow the diet suggested in this book. It is especially important to eat plenty of fresh, raw fruits and vegetables; drink plenty of water and herbal teas; and eat a lot of protein, particularly vegetable proteins such as beans and seeds, but try to limit dairy proteins.

NATURAL REMEDIES

In addition to the above, there is also a whole range of natural and herbal medicines that are used to enhance the immune system. These include echinacea, garlic, ginger, goldenseal, aloe vera, mushrooms, elderberry, and many others. Many appear to be very effective, but first make sure that you are getting all the nutrients you need. Once any nutritional deficiencies are sorted out, you can then move on to herbal remedies.

CHAPTER 6

Neurological Disorders

OUR BRAINS ARE THE MOST important part of our bodies—they make us who and what we are. They control everything we do and say, and their health is fundamental to our survival. Unfortunately the massive recent escalation of brain-related health problems suggests that there is something about modern living that has quite literally poisoned our minds.

In the past, scientists have tried to explain this massive increase in disease by blaming an aging population. However, people are getting these illnesses at an ever-younger age, and this fact, coupled with a dramatic rise in childhood brain diseases such as autism, suggests that other influences are causing our brains to malfunction.

Clues can be found by looking to our new environment. If you consider that a sizable 25 percent of the thousands of chemicals released into our environment are known neurotoxins (nerve-poisoning chemicals) and that our children are increasingly being bombarded with these development-damaging toxins, this increase in brain disease starts to make sense. If you put this together with the fact that our brains are being starved of the nutrients they need, it should come as no surprise that all sorts of brain diseases are on the increase.

Common Neurological Disorders Associated with Chemical Exposure

Autism

Behavioral problems

Brain cancer

Dementia

Depression

Dyslexia and other learning disorders

Epilepsy

Memory loss

Multiple sclerosis

Parkinson's disease

Schizophrenia

The good news is that we can do a lot both to improve the current situation and to prevent these diseases from happening in the first place. To find out why our brain and nervous system is so sensitive to toxins and nutrient deficiencies, we need to understand more about what the brain is and how it works.

What Makes Our Nervous System So Vulnerable to Chemical Toxins?

Although our brains are able to control our bodies remarkably well, they are like sitting ducks when it comes to their ability to defend themselves from the raft of toxic chemicals they are now exposed to on a daily basis.

How Do I Know If I Am Being Affected by These Toxins?

The range of symptoms and signs of dysfunction people experience from brain-damaging toxins can be very wide ranging and include the following:

Anxiety

Balance problems

Behavioral problems

Collapse

Deafness and visual problems

Depression

Dizziness

General weakness and fatigue

Headache

Impaired concentration

Learning difficulties

Memory defects

Migraines

Movement difficulties

Panic attacks

Paralysis

Reduced dexterity

Reduced intelligence

Seizures

Sensation of pins and needles

Skin numbness

Speech difficulties

Suicidal tendencies

The excellent blood supply the brain receives means that it is exposed to a higher level of blood-borne toxins, while its high fatty content means that it acts as a sponge—soaking up the large number of fat-loving toxins in the blood. Once these chemicals arrive at the brain, they quickly take up residence and are then very hard to shift. Not only is the blood-brain barrier unable to prevent these modern artificial chemicals from entering, these chemicals can also make the barrier much less effective, allowing more chemicals and other unwanted substances to enter.

Once in the brain, they are comparatively harder to neutralize or remove. One reason is the comparatively lower level of antioxidant nutrients present in the brain. This means that there are fewer antioxidants present to neutralize the higher levels of tissue-damaging free radicals triggered by the presence of these artificial toxic chemicals. This, in combination with the smaller number of defense mechanisms present in brain tissue and our poor, less-nutritious diets, magnifies the amount of damage chemicals can wreak.

Added to this is the fact that nerve cells appear to be very delicate creatures. Unlike most other parts of our bodies, once damaged, our brains are not able to regenerate themselves. Many toxic chemicals are highly effective nerve poisons, which, in addition to killing nerve cells outright, can also prevent growing brains from developing properly and can damage normal levels of neurotransmitters and hormones.

The end result is that this continuous poisoning by toxins, in conjunction with increasingly poor diet, appears to be a major factor behind the growing number of people affected by brain diseases.

Memory Loss: Clearing the Brain Fog

If you ever have trouble remembering a name or lose your train of thought in the middle of a sentence, you may be experiencing brain fog. Brain fog sufferers usually have one or more of the following symptoms: forgetfulness, spaciness, feelings of confusion, and inability to focus. This is a major problem in today's dog-eat-dog world, where being alert and having a good memory are vital. Memory loss can cause major ripples throughout the rest of your life and may potentially result in permanent memory loss, taking the form of dementia.

Unfortunately, poor memory and concentration are becoming more and more commonplace. The number of people suffering from officially recognized memory-loss diseases such as Alzheimer's or other forms of dementia is very much on the rise. The number of people expected to develop full-blown dementia is expected to more than double by the middle of the twenty-first century. But unlike diseases such as full-blown dementia, a poor memory is not treated as a separate condition for which there are well-known treatments. Consequently it tends not to be taken seriously as a "real" problem—most doctors are simply not able to deal with it.

The fact that so many chemicals are known to possess widespread brain-damaging actions will lead you to appreciate that our increasing exposure to chemicals could be a major factor underlying brain fog and dementia. Because thinking requires complex activity among many different parts of the brain, damage to one part can effect the level of overall brain functioning. In fact, brain fog is often one of the first signs of a recognizable sensitivity to toxic chemicals.

Many pesticides are powerful nerve agents. Indeed, one of the most commonly used groups of pesticides, known as organophosphates, were originally created as nerve agents and used in World War II. After this, they started to be used on crops as pesticides. They made highly effective bug killers, poisoning the nervous system and rapidly paralyzing the pest/bug to stop it from breathing or moving. Organophosphates

Toxins Known to Target Memory

Pesticides (most types)

Solvents

Toxic metals

are now commonly found on our food and in many other nonfood products such as household fly sprays.

Organophosphates are also used by terrorist groups and other organizations as chemical warfare weapons. For instance, they were used by the Iraqi army on the Kurds and in the Tokyo subway terrorist attack. The survivors of the Tokyo attack (and the people sent to help them) experienced long-term memory loss as a result of exposure to these chemicals. And the greater the exposure, the more severe the memory loss. However, despite their known ability to cause memory loss and poison the nervous system, organophosphates have played an extremely controversial role in the treatment of dementia.

You may be surprised to discover that organophosphates had actually been used in clinical trials to "treat" patients with Alzheimer's disease. In this role they are not referred to as organophosphates, but were described as anticholinesterases. The organophosphate used for this purpose, known as metrifonate, is converted into a chemical called dichlorvos, once it's in the body. Dichlorvos is what is known as the active metabolite and is thought to be largely responsible for the "therapeutic effect." (Dichlorvos has recently been banned in the UK and removed from all insect-killing preparations such as household sprays because of a cancer alert; it is still in use in America.) Despite getting approval for treatment of Alzheimer's, following a number of drug trials, this substance is not currently in use, although other chemicals with similar actions are.

Next, let us consider solvents, the highly fat-soluble liquids that are commonly used as anesthetics. Solvents have powerful mind-altering actions and are strongly linked with causing not only brain fog but Alzheimer's itself. A study carried out by Dr. Walter Kukull, Professor of Epidemiology, University of Washington School of Public Health and Community Medicine, found that people who had worked with organic solvents, such as benzene, toluene, phenols, alcohols, and ketones in the past were more at risk of developing Alzheimer's disease.

Finally, people who have Alzheimer's disease have been found to have higher levels of certain metals in their brains and in their bloodstream, including substances such as aluminum, mercury, iron, and copper. Higher levels of metals end up being stored in brain tissue than should be there due to the brain's inability to handle these substances. Other people with memory problems include workers exposed to higher levels of lead—as the greater the lead exposure, the greater the memory loss.

By generally lowering your exposure to chemical toxins and by starting a suitable detox program, you can do your bit to both de-fog your brain and lower your odds of developing a more severe memory-loss problem in the future.

Natural Highs: Beating Blues

Despite the obvious benefits to our everyday lives that modern-day living brings in the form of electric lighting and a highly sophisticated communications network, the stress accompanying this round-the-clock lifestyle appears to be decreasing our ability to enjoy life to the full. If you combine this with our ever-increasing use of mood-altering substances such as stimulants, alcohol, prescription medications, and drugs; our increased exposure to toxic chemicals; and our decreased intake of mood-stabilizing nutrients as a result of our overly processed and less nutritious diet—then the risk of developing a mood disturbance increases still further.

It is, therefore, hardly surprising that moderate or severe depression is now one of the most common diseases of our time, affecting nearly 3 percent. And that figure is thought to greatly underestimate the real numbers since only one third of sufferers ever receive treatment.

Although all of us at some stage experience periods of intense sadness, true depression can be completely overwhelming and totally disabling, causing the affected person to effectively withdraw from participating in everyday life. True depression affects people in different ways, with symptoms ranging from increased anxiety to overpowering feelings of hopelessness and suicidal thoughts. Some people with manic depression (otherwise known as bipolar disease) have periods of low mood interspersed with periods of tremendous elation, known as mania, in which their thinking processes are clearly disturbed.

These powerful feelings are thought to be caused by imbalances in the level of mood-enhancing natural substances known as neurotransmitters, such as catecholamines, serotonin, and other substances. These are our "happy hormones." In fact, the main conventional drugs targeted at alleviating depression are thought to work by artificially boosting or interfering with our level of these neurotransmitters.

Since approximately 90 percent of the most common types of toxic chemicals in our food and environment are known to alter levels of happy hormones, it is not surprising that the link between toxic chemicals and depression is very strong. Indeed, considering the sheer number of chemicals known to damage mood-controlling hormones, it seems incredible that this connection has been virtually ignored by not only conventional medicine, but to some extent by alternative medicine as well.

Common Symptoms of Depression

Disturbed eating, sleeping, and bowel habits

Excessive weight loss or weight gain

Feeling worse in the morning

Inability to concentrate

Inability to enjoy anything in life

Increased anxiety

Low self-esteem

Overpowering feelings of hopelessness and suicidal thoughts

Sleep disturbance—normally waking up early in the morning

A tendency to burst into tears

How Chemicals Cause Depression

The most obvious way of illustrating this link is to look at people who use chemicals on a regular basis, for example farmers and other people working with pesticides. People in this group not only have higher rates of depression, they are also more likely to commit suicide. But it's not just pesticide workers who are at risk, as others can also be affected. Over a two-year period ending in 1996, the organophosphate pesticide known as methyl parathion was sprayed by unlicensed pest-control operators in more than 1,500 homes and offices. Over half of the victims interviewed reported depressive symptoms at levels suggesting probable clinical depression.

Toxic metals, such as mercury, lead, and vanadium, appear to be another major source of depression-causing substances. For example, people with mercury poisoning symptoms from their amalgam fillings also had a higher rate of mental strain and higher depressive scores than normal. Another study showed that the removal of mercury fillings resulted in improvements in 70 percent of those who suffered from mercury-linked

Chemicals Known to Be Linked to Depression

Environmental pollutants

Pesticides (a classic example are organophosphates)

Prescription drugs in the following classes: barbiturates, tranquilizers, sleeping pills, heart drugs that contain reserpine, beta-blockers, high-blood-pressure drugs, ulcer drugs, systemic corticosteroids, anticonvulsants, anti-parkinsonism drugs, antibiotics, and certain painkillers and arthritis drugs

Solvents

Toxic metals (mercury, lead, antimony)

health problems, which included depression. Lead is another toxic metal known to cause depression. This can be clearly seen in metal foundry workers who are exposed to lead in their jobs. When their blood levels of lead were measured, it became clear that the higher the lead levels, the greater the levels of depression. Those with higher levels of lead in their body also had a greater degree of other mood-related problems.

Another very common group of mood-altering substances we are all in contact with as part of our everyday lives is solvents, with alcohol being perhaps the best-known brain depressant. Of a group of people who have had a greater exposure to solvents as part of their work, 50 percent had evidence of mood disorders including depression. But again it's not just people who work with chemicals who are in the firing line, as the simple act of self-medication with an insect repellent solvent commonly known as DEET (N,N-diethyl-m-toluamide) can trigger manic depression.

Many prescription drugs made of synthetic chemicals are known to cause imbalances in the brain's happy hormones. Consequently dozens of drugs used to control blood pressure and treat heart-rate problems and infections can also trigger depression, because in lowering the levels of catecholamines and serotonin to treat the health problem, they have in effect created a new one. These drugs are becoming so widespread that some scientists think that the general increases in depression rates could be partly due to the increased use of these medications.

Indeed, as many pesticides found in our foods are made of similar chemicals to those used as catecholamine-altering prescription medicines, you could be unknowingly exposed to these same mood-depressing chemicals just by eating conventionally grown foods.

By lowering your body burdens of the above by going on a detox program and by limiting your future contact with toxins, you can do a great deal to increase your own natural ability to banish the blues.

Parkinson's Disease

When the ever-youthful Michael J. Fox developed Parkinson's disease (PD), public perception of this disease changed overnight. Far from being confined to older people, this illness was now seen to affect people in their prime of life. The revival in interest in this disease resulted in the uncomfortable discovery that the characteristics of Parkinson's have been changing over recent years, so much so that the age at which people develop Parkinson's disease has dramatically fallen.

In fact, in the space of a couple of decades, a totally new group of people with PD has emerged: those who develop PD before the age of forty. Further investigation revealed that people in this younger group tended to have a higher exposure to environmental chemicals, such as insecticides, from living in a fumigated house or in an agricultural area. Their disease also tended to be more aggressive than that seen in older people, which is particularly distressing in view of the fact that there is currently no known cure.

Parkinson's disease is a neuro-degenerative disorder, or wasting brain disease. Two hundred years ago it was very rare, but now it is the second most common neuro-degenerative disorder, affecting 1 percent of people over sixty years old. For some reason, nerve cells that produce the neurotransmitter known as dopamine start dying in the part of the brain that controls movement, known as the substantia nigra. As the number of nerve cells decreases, so does the ability of the remaining nerves to make sufficient amounts of dopamine.

This is a problem because dopamine production in this part of the brain plays a major role both in initiating and controlling our body movements. The subsequent low levels of dopamine help to explain the muscular symptoms characteristic of PD, such as tremor, muscle rigidity, and a generally reduced level of movement. Unfortunately, once this process starts, it appears to be progressive.

Current methods of treatment tend to be based on prescription medications. However, while they can help initially, they tend to become less and less effective with time. In addition they also have their fair share of side effects, some of which can be debilitating. Although there are surgical methods being developed to treat Parkinson's disease, at present they are very much in their infancy.

Parkinson's disease differs from parkinsonism. Parkinsonism has many of the muscular features of Parkinson's disease, but symptoms are known to be caused by other factors such as drugs, viral diseases, Wilson's disease (an inherited disorder that causes excessive amounts of copper to accumulate in the body), brain tumors, toxic-metal exposure, environmental toxins, and trauma. Consequently, more people suffer with parkinsonism than Parkinson's disease.

CHEMICALS AND PARKINSON'S DISEASE

To date there are many things known to trigger Parkinson's, but out of all the known or suspected factors, exposure to toxic chemicals ranks as one of the highest. Not only has a previous exposure to toxic chemicals been found in those developing Parkinson's disease at an earlier age, it also increases the risk of developing it at an older age. Chemical poisoning can produce many of the symptoms experienced by PD and can also trigger the disease itself. Indeed, some chemicals are so effective in triggering parkinsonism that they are used to create animal models of this disease for research purposes.

One of these is a synthetic chemical created in the 1980s known as MPTP (1-methyl-4-phenyl-1,2,3,6-tetrahydropyridine). It was found to be a potential dopaminergic neurotoxin following the observation that humans accidentally exposed to this chemical developed irreversible clinical, chemical, and pathological alterations mimicing those found in Parkinson's disease. Since then, this chemical has been used to reproduce an almost perfect model of parkinsonism in animals.

The problem we now face is that substances containing MPTP-like fragments are used as herbicides, drugs, and intermediates in the synthesis of many artificial compounds, including some drugs. Our increased exposure to MPTP-like pesticides and contaminants is thought to be one of the reasons behind the recent increase in Parkinson's disease. Indeed, in the light of the extensive body of research which shows so many other toxic chemicals that particularly target and lower the production of dopamine (one of the happy hormones so universally damaged by chemicals), it becomes more surprising that more people are *not* developing Parkinson's disease.

The chemicals implicated can be guessed at by looking at the people who tend to get Parkinson's disease. Farmers and agricultural workers working with pesticides are at higher risk, as are toxic-metal workers.

Exposure to toxins at an ever-earlier age tends to weaken the body's systems, and the number and levels of chemicals in our environment is increasing. These factors work in combination to increase the adult susceptibility to these pesticides, increasing the damage they can do. Those less able to deal with chemical toxins and who have a less-developed detoxification process appear to be the most vulnerable.

This increasing sensitivity to chemicals could be why more and more younger people are developing PD. Not only are people who work with chemicals at risk, but anyone who is exposed to larger amounts of these chemicals in their everyday life is increasingly at risk. This increased sensitivity to chemicals could ultimately result in chemicals initiating reactions that result in the destruction of the brain cells in the substantia nigra.

While PD tends to be progressive once it has developed, you can see from the above that it makes sense to avoid and rid the body of chemi-

Chemical Causes of Parkinson's Disease and Parkinsonism

Drinking well water (probably related to the water contaminants)

Drugs (e.g., reserpine, phenothiazine, butyrophenones)

Herbicides (like paraquat and rotenone)

Organochlorines

Organophosphates

Pesticides known as synthetic pyrethroids

Toxic metal exposure (aluminum, copper, iron, cobalt, manganese, lead, mercury)

cals that speed up the destruction of the remaining dopamine-producing nerve cells in the substantia nigra. In addition to reducing the chance of developing PD and parkinsonism, this should have the effect of slowing down disease progression and maximizing the body's natural production of dopamine.

Multiple Sclerosis

Multiple sclerosis (MS) affects more than one in 2,000 of the population in many developed countries and is one of the commonest neurological causes of long-term disability. And there are no signs of the problem abating as the number of people being diagnosed with this disease has more than doubled in recent years.

MS can affect any part of the body, but the most commonly reported symptoms are double or blurred vision in one or both eyes, pins and needles in the extremities, slurred speech, difficulty in walking, dragging either foot, loss of coordination and balance, and loss of sensation anywhere in the body.

The clinical progression characteristically involves relapsing and remitting episodes when the symptoms get worse, then improve. The symptoms and signs of the first attack usually fade within one to three months and after a variable interval there may be a recurrence. Other people never lose their original symptoms and continue to deteriorate. Although the main problem originates from damage to the myelin sheath (the thin protective layer of fatty membrane that surrounds the nerve tracts in the brain and spinal cord), symptoms vary widely, and the term "multiple sclerosis" is now thought to cover a collection of quite disparate problems.

The myelin sheath acts like the insulation around electrical wires, allowing the current—or in the case of the human body, the neurological signals—to travel through without loss of power and strength. Any damage to this protective layer can cause the electrical signal to "leak" and so lose power and become distorted.

In MS, this damage is caused by inflammation, making the sheath lose some of its covering, a process known as demyelination. Hard scar tissue then forms over these damaged patches or lesions and multiple sclerosis (literally "many scars") is the result. These patches of demyelination (known as plaques) can occur anywhere, which explains the wide-ranging symptoms experienced by people with MS.

The entire gamut of toxic chemicals and other factors in our environment appears to conspire to slowly poison our nervous systems. Although MS has a very strong genetic component, there is growing evidence that our environment is playing a vitally important role in the triggering and development of MS.

How Chemicals Are Linked to MS

The evidence that MS may be some sort of toxic overload from man-made poisons started to arise following "outbreaks" of MS that occurred following local cases of environmental pollution with toxic

Chemicals Linked to Multiple Sclerosis

Artificial sweeteners such as aspartame (in diet, low sugar, and sugar-free products)

Low-level radiation

Medications

Organochlorines

Overuse of antibiotics

Pesticides

Solvents

Synthetic chemicals

Toxic metal poisoning (particularly mercury)

Vaccinations

metals. One of these episodes occurred in Key West, Florida, between 1983 and 1985, when thirty to forty people developed MS. This was eventually traced to the dumping of toxic debris containing high levels of mercury and lead.

What makes this link with mercury more compelling is that the mass hepatitis B vaccination in France (mercury was used as it is commonly used in vaccines as a preservative) triggered an outbreak of hundreds of cases of MS. Another common source of mercury is amalgam, so it may not be too surprising to hear that the health of MS patients can significantly improve after mercury fillings have been replaced with a less-toxic, nonmetallic substitute.

Solvents also appear to be strongly linked to MS as those working with these substances have a greater risk of developing this disease. Those particularly at risk are painters, construction workers, and food processing workers. There is also evidence that people with MS have higher levels of solvents in their bodies, possibly as a result of higher levels of exposure or a relative inability to process and expel these chemicals, which are highly fat soluble and damage the nerve sheath.

Like most other chronic diseases, MS occurrence is linked to pesticides, in particular the highly fat-soluble organochlorine pesticides. In one academic paper, a man with no previous medical complaints developed neurological symptoms characteristic of MS after being exposed to organochlorine pesticides on just two occasions. These symptoms progressed until his death. At autopsy, his brain showed classical findings of multiple sclerosis. Interestingly, people with MS tend to have more than double the types of organochlorine pesticides in their bodies than those without MS.

The fact is that MS patients have up to five times the overall number of artificial chemicals in their bodies as healthy people do. This suggests that in addition to being exposed to more-toxic chemicals, people who develop chemically linked MS are less able to process and expel these chemicals, and so they end up accumulating in the body. This relative inability to process toxins may derive from many things, including a genetic inability to detoxify, as well as increased exposure to chemicals and poor nutrition. By reducing your future exposure to chemicals and by embarking on a good detox program, you may not only help reduce existing symptoms and the number of relapses, you can also reduce the risk of developing this debilitating disease in the future.

Maximizing Brain and Nervous System Health

The Toxic Overload program will lower the body's exposure to nerve-damaging chemical toxins and give your body the nutrients it needs to remove the most toxic brain-damaging chemicals. By lowering your future exposure to chemicals you will not only minimize any further damage, but also reduce your chances of developing another chemical-related brain disease.

You can never start too soon in avoiding brain-damaging toxins as the earlier appropriate treatment is started, the less likely that early problems, such as memory loss, will end up progressing into a permanent disease such as dementia. Even if diseases have already developed, by knowing what makes things worse it is sometimes possible to slow down disease progression and even alleviate certain devastating symptoms.

SUPPLEMENTS

The program in chapter 2 will not only ensure that your nervous system gets the nutrients it needs to clean up and kick out large amounts of brain-damaging toxins, but also enough to optimize brain functioning.

Essential oils play a vital role in brain health as over half the fats in our brains are made up of polyunsaturated fat. However, these fats, commonly found in raw nuts, seeds, and fish, are becoming more and more of a rarity in our diets. Consequently, this lack of fat, particularly omega-3s, can damage the fundamental way our brain is designed to work, making it much more prone not only to chemical damage, but to virtually all forms of brain and nerve diseases such as depression, MS, developmental disorders (autism, dyslexia, and ADHD), Parkinson's disease, and dementia. This is why supplementation of this nutrient is so important.

Due to the constant level of activity going on in processing information and controlling body functions, our brains have a high need for other nutrients such as vitamins and minerals. This is why all of the above brain or nervous system disorders, such as depression, memory loss, dementia, Parkinson's disease, and all the childhood developmental disorders, are more common in those who are deficient in one or more essential nutrient.

Antioxidants not only prevent toxin-induced brain damage, but they can also lower the future possibility of getting Alzheimer's and other brain diseases. Antioxidants that are particularly beneficial for preventing Alzheimer's include vitamins C and E, selenium, alpha-lipoic acid, glutathione, and N-acetylcysteine. Low levels of these nutrients not only make the brain more vulnerable to damage from toxic chemicals, but also lower or distort the levels of neurotransmitters or brain hormones, which are vital to the regular functioning of the brain.

Lack of other nutrients, such as vitamins B_6, B_{12}, and folic acid, is known to cause blood vessel disease. As a good blood flow is important to ensure that the brain gets enough nutrients, people low in these nutrients tend to have a greater degree of blood vessel disease and a higher incidence of mild memory loss, age-related memory loss, vascular dementia, and Alzheimer's disease. In addition to this, many prescription medications can also induce certain nutrient deficiencies that increase the risk of depression still further. For instance, the contraceptive pill is known to deplete the body of many essential nutrients such as vitamin B_6, and low levels of this vitamin are strongly linked to depression. The minerals zinc and magnesium appear to play a vital role in enhancing brain functioning, particularly behavioral problems such as depression and ADHD (see chapter 13).

Higher levels of supplements appear to offer dramatic benefits in treating different forms of depression. A study was carried out at the University of Calgary, Alberta, Canada, based on giving people who suffered from manic depression higher levels of vitamin and mineral supplementation. Their findings were astonishing. For those who completed the minimum six-month open trial, symptom reduction ranged from 55 percent to 66 percent, and their need for the appropriate prescription antidepressant medications decreased by more than 50 percent. In some cases, the supplement replaced antidepressant medications and the patients remained well.

Not only will a good nutritional program tackle diseases and their causes, but it can also have other benefits such as improved intelligence and behavior. For example, most children's diets are low in nutrients, so giving them vitamins and minerals could improve their schoolwork. Other studies show that young people in prison commit 35 percent fewer violent offenses after just two weeks of getting a good level of vitamins, minerals, and essential fats. The bottom line is that you have to give the brain what it needs if you want it to work properly, and if you don't, you can't be too surprised if things go wrong.

DIET

To cleanse your body of unwanted toxins and encourage optimum brain function, follow the diet suggested in chapter 3. It is especially important to eat plenty of fresh and raw fruits and vegetables, drink plenty of water and herbal teas, and eat a lot of foods rich in omega-3 oils.

NATURAL REMEDIES

In addition to the above, there is also a whole range of natural and herbal medicines that can be used to enhance the nervous system. Many appear to be very effective, such as ginkgo biloba extract for memory loss and Saint-John's-wort for depression. First make sure that you are getting all the nutrients, and once any nutritional deficiencies have been sorted out, then move on to herbal remedies. I would also advise anyone starting with these remedies, particularly Saint-John's-wort, to do so under the supervision of a trained herbalist, as it has been linked to side effects such as sensitivity to light.

CHAPTER 7

Digestive Disorders

WE ALL KNOW THAT YOU are what you eat. So if your diet is full of nutritionally deficient foods, you will eventually end up paying the price in faulty digestion, poor absorption, intestine infections, bloating, and inflammation. However, few people realize that many so-called healthy foods, such as salmon, apples, and strawberries, could also be damaging your intestines. The main problem doesn't lie with the foods themselves, but rather in the level of chemicals they contain.

Agriculture has changed so dramatically over the past one hundred years that some of the foods previously considered the healthiest are the most contaminated with artificial chemicals. Unfortunately, when we eat these contaminated foods, the chemicals that enter our digestive system poison any part of it that they subsequently come into contact with. This is because the toxic effects of these chemicals don't conveniently turn off once eaten. Worse still, these food-borne chemicals will also not yet have had a chance to be processed and neutralized to some extent by the liver, consequently they are likely to be even more dangerous (see chapter 3).

Because of this, our digestive systems are directly in the firing line of food-borne toxins. In addition to which, our stomachs also get exposed to toxic metals, such as mercury from dental fillings and aluminum from food additives, food preservatives, colorings, pesticides, solvents, and a whole number of other pollutants. On top of this, our digestive system also has to face the existing background levels that all the rest of the body tissues now have to contend with.

The problem is, our digestive system and the tissues that control it, such as the brain, hormones, nerves, and all the other major digestive organs such as the liver and the pancreas, are all extremely vulnerable to chemical damage. Chemicals have been shown to damage the digestive system by:

➤ Damaging the inner wall of the stomach, reducing the overall ability to absorb essential nutrients and vitamins and minerals from food.

➤ Triggering inflammation in the bowel wall.

➤ Destroying nutrients, such as vitamins, which are present in the stomach.

➤ Increasing or reducing production of digestive juices and digestive hormones. A reduction can result in undigested foods and overproduction can result in ulceration.

➤ Reducing the thickness of the protective mucous layer protecting the bowel wall from powerful digestive juices, thereby increasing the risk of ulceration.

➤ Killing many of the good bacteria in the gut, upsetting the balance and making it easier for "bad" bugs to multiply. This could result in ulceration and infections such as thrush. Bacterial imbalance can also affect food breakdown and the ability of bacteria to produce essential vitamins.

➤ Damaging the parts of the brain and the hormones that control digestion.

➤ Poisoning the underlying immune system, which increases the chances of developing an underlying food allergy or intolerance.

➤ Making the muscles in the bowel wall either go into spasm (causing cramps and diarrhea) or to relax (leading to excessive dilation and constipation).

➤ Exposing the gut to significant amounts of cancer-causing chemicals.

Digestive Problems Associated with Chemicals

Bad breath

Burning of the tongue and mouth

Celiac disease

Colitis

Diseases of the colon and rectum

Dry mouth

Food absorption disorders

Gastric and duodenal ulceration

Gastritis

Heartburn

Hemorrhoids

Irritable bowel syndrome

Leukoplakia

Mouth ulcers

Pruritus ani

Regional enteritis

Stomach cancer

This extensive ability of chemicals to damage our digestive system could help explain why the number of people with digestive disorders has substantially increased over the last few decades.

Food Intolerances

Something in our current environment is making us react to foods we could previously tolerate, which is why the number of people with certain types of food intolerances, such as peanut allergies, has doubled in some populations every six years, despite a steady level of peanut consumption. The reason why we are starting to react to our food is challenging many scientists. However, Dr. Claudia Millar from the University of Texas Health Science Center at San Antonio has published a very interesting academic paper that provides a credible explanation. She has suggested that the rise in food intolerances could be due to an early exposure to chemical toxins such as pesticides, solvents, and indoor air contaminants: people who are more exposed to these substances are much more likely to react to foods that they could previously tolerate. So what are the different types of food intolerances?

Nonallergic and lactose intolerance reactions make up the largest group of those suffering from food intolerances. The most common symptom of this type of food intolerance is a skin rash. But digestive symptoms, such as diarrhea, constipation, and stomach cramps, and in some cases breathing difficulties, can also occur. These varied reactions themselves arise from a variety of different problems with food digestion, absorption, or metabolism. Food intolerances can be lessened by identifying the food the body is reacting to, such as milk, then removing it from the diet. Lactose intolerance is an inability to breakdown one of the sugars in cow's milk. A deficiency of this enzyme is often inherited, and there is a strong association with the disorder and certain ethnic groups. Prevalence among Asian populations is nearly 100 percent, 80 percent among Native Americans, and 70 percent among African Americans. Only 20 percent of the Caucasian population is lactose intolerant. While the genetic component of lactose intolerance is strong, more and more people are developing this problem during late childhood and adulthood.

There is evidence that food allergies are caused by an immunological reaction. This type of intolerance is thought to affect a minority of those with food intolerances. However, due to the often severe allergic reaction to certain foods, such as peanuts, nuts, and eggs, they make up an important group. Symptoms of food allergy in children are diverse and include vomiting, poor weight gain, abdominal pain, malabsorption of nutrients, coughing, wheezing, rhinitis (dripping nose), atopic eczema, hives, and angioedema (swelling of mucous membranes or organs due to an allergic reaction).

Pseudoallergic reactions to food tend to be triggered by chemicals in and around food products, for instance colorings, preservatives, flavorings, and additives. Although the types of symptoms brought about can overlap with those of true food allergies, the mechanisms that bring them about differ. Avoidance of these additives is the best management tool.

Celiac disease is yet another example of a food intolerance. It arises when the body reacts to a component known as gluten, commonly found in wheat, barley, rye, and oats. This disease tends to reveal itself in early childhood when affected infants fail to thrive, develop anemia, have pale bowel movements, and develop a swollen abdomen. Treatment involves eliminating gluten from the diet as much as possible for life, which, as you can imagine, proves a great hardship for all those affected.

How Chemicals Trigger or Exacerbate Food Intolerances

Toxic chemicals are thought to be involved in food intolerance reactions in two main ways, by:

➤ Damaging the underlying immune system, making it overreact to substances it could previously tolerate.
➤ Directly triggering food intolerance reactions.

Chemical damage to the immune system is a well-known consequence of chemical overexposure. The ability of chemicals to excessively stimulate the immune system, making it overreact to substances, such as foods, that it could previously tolerate, appears to be common (see chapter 5).

Although damage to the underlying immune system appears to be happening in all forms of food intolerances, the exact form of food intolerance developed will depend on many different factors, such as the type of chemical involved, the body's genetic makeup, and the body's general nutritional state.

Chemicals Associated with Immune Disorders

Chlorine in drinking water and swimming pools

Cigarette smoke

Drugs (such as aspirin, antibiotics, painkillers, and insect repellents)

Environmental pollutants (dioxins, PCBs)

Fluoride in water and dental treatments

Fluorine and chlorine

Food preservatives, colorings, and other additives

Latex rubber

Pesticides (particularly synthetic pyrethroids, organophosphates, carbamates, and organochlorines)

Plastics (including bisphenol A)

Solvents (such as formaldehyde and xylene)

Sunscreens, perfumes, and other toiletry components

Surgical prosthetic implants

Toxic metals (e.g., mercury and aluminum)

Wood preservatives

Chemicals also directly trigger food intolerance reactions. In this way food colorings, additives, flavorings, fragrances, and preservatives are thought to bring about pseudoallergic food intolerance reactions.

This strong link between chemicals and food intolerances suggests that a reduction in the overall body burden of chemicals from food and other sources would result in a considerable benefit in all types of food intolerance reactions. Not only would this reduce the number of people who develop these reactions, it would also ease the symptoms of those affected by all forms of food intolerances.

In addition to cutting down on one's general exposure to chemicals, it would also make sense to embark on a long-term detox program designed to effectively tackle the existing chemical body burden.

Inflammatory Bowel Disease

Many hundreds of thousands of people around the world every year are now touched by inflammatory bowel disease (IBD). With one Scottish study showing a threefold rise in childhood Crohn's disease between 1968 and 1983, and a recent follow-up revealing further rises, it appears to be one of those chronic illnesses that is very much on the increase.

According to conventional medicine, inflammatory bowel disease is an incurable condition, the cause of which is as yet unknown. However, evidence is building that IBD is brought about by a combination of genetic and environmental factors, such as toxic chemicals.

But whatever the trigger, the overriding opinion is that IBD is autoimmune in nature. At the heart of the problem is a malfunctioning immune system, which for some reason is sent into overdrive, and as a result attacks and inflames the body's own tissues (see chapter 5). This is reflected in the fact that the majority of conventional treatments are targeted at suppressing the immune system. However, while these drugs can often suppress the disease, they do not alter the overall long-term prognosis, very probably because they fail to tackle whatever it is that causes the imbalanced and malfunctioning immune system in the first place. Determining the factors that cause this immune system chaos probably holds the key to solving the IBD mystery.

For diagnostic purposes, doctors tend to divide IBD into two categories: Crohn's disease and ulcerative colitis (UC). Crohn's involves all the layers of tissue in the bowel and can affect any part of the gastrointestinal tract from the mouth to the anus, while ulcerative colitis affects only the colon or rectum. Despite this superficial division, there is a compelling argument that Crohn's and UC represent two different poles of the same disease. This is because of the marked similarity between these two conditions, reflected in the fact that no single test is sufficient to diagnose either disease. Indeed, in 10 to 20 percent of cases it is almost impossible to differentiate between the two.

CHEMICALS AND INFLAMMATORY BOWEL DISEASE

The first clue as to what could be underlying this hyperactive immune system syndrome came about with the timing of the discovery of IBD, as it was first described in 1913, approximately a decade or two after synthetic chemicals were first developed. This is highly relevant, as in retrospect we now know that many toxic chemicals have the ability to unbalance the whole immune system, increasing our propensity to develop autoimmune diseases. Indeed, some synthetic chemicals are so good at this—for example, a chemical called trinitrobenzene sulfonic—that they are actually used to induce an animal model of inflammatory bowel disease.

Many chemicals are known to trigger IBD (see sidebar, page 162). When an already chemically damaged and therefore weakened system is exposed to a high level of one of the following toxins, or a combination of chemicals with other digestive system stressors, the balance is tipped, resulting in the development of disease. In other words, the ultimate responsibility probably lies with a combination of chemicals and other factors rather than with just one factor alone.

Those who have an increased intake of aluminum in the form of food additives and colorants tend to have an increased chance of developing Crohn's disease. Furthermore, when these additives are cut out

Chemicals That Trigger or Exacerbate Inflammatory Bowel Disease

Additives in carbonated beverages (the preservative benzoic acid)

Chemicals found in cigarettes

Conventional medicines (antibiotics, nonsteroidal anti-inflammatories, the contraceptive pill, gold, and sulphasalazine)

Fluoride

Pollution from urban living

Preservatives and food additives

Solvents (such as benzene)

Synthetic chemicals

Toxic metals (such as the aluminum and mercury in vaccines)

Vaccinations

of the diet, symptoms of Crohn's are significantly improved. As urban living and vaccinations expose us to greater amounts of aluminum, this could partly explain the observed link between the urban diet and Crohn's disease.

Other chemicals known to be associated with Crohn's include some of those found in cigarette smoke, such as benzene, cadmium, arsenic, nickel, chromium, 2-naphthyl-amine, vinyl chloride, 4-aminobiphenyl, and beryllium. The increase of free radicals induced by exposure of the gut to cigarette smoke has been shown to increase the allergic and inflammatory response of the bowel.

Part of the reason why cigarette smoke is so strongly linked to IBD could be due to the presence of the chemical benzene, since benzene is found in the chemical actually used to trigger IBD in animals in order to create an experimental model. Unfortunately, benzene is also commonly found in most carbonated drinks, as the preservative benzoic acid. So our huge consumption of sodas could be contributing to the rising incidence of IBD. Benzoic acid is also used as a preservative and antioxidant most frequently in fruit products, such as pickled produce and salad dressings and bottled sauces. Sodium benzoate, a salt of benzoic acid, is another common chemical preservative to look out for on food labels and avoid.

So many chemicals present in our bodies, such as pesticides, toxic metals, plastics, and solvents, among many others, can also fundamentally damage the immune system by overactivating it and triggering long-term chronic inflammation, which could also be a contributing factor (see page 164).

Due to the role that chemicals play in triggering IBD, it would be a sensible move to lower our daily exposure to these autoimmune-triggering chemicals, as well as to improve the body's ability to shift its existing chemical load.

Irritable Bowel Syndrome

Irritable bowel syndrome appears to be one of the most common health problems in the world. In the United States up to one in five people suffer from this condition, and if you suffer from a general range of bowel problems that don't fall under any neat category, chances are that you may have irritable bowel syndrome. Because this term is applied to a spectrum of complaints, there is no agreed precise definition of what IBS is. Because of this lack of clarity, this condition is often known by several other names, such as spastic colon, mucus colitis, or noninflammatory bowel disease.

Those affected by IBS usually have variable periods of relapse and remission. Common symptoms include bloating, abdominal pain, gas, alternating diarrhea and constipation, excess mucus, an urgency to defecate, and indigestion. But before a diagnosis of IBS can be made, you must be tested for other bowel diseases that have similar symptoms. IBS is a so

Chemical Triggers of IBS

Chemical fumes (such as those from perfumes, paints, new carpet, and automobile exhaust)

Chlorine

Environmental pollution (such as auto exhaust)

Pesticides (particularly organochlorines)

Solvents (such as formaldehyde, phenol, and ethanol)

Toxic metals

called "disease of exclusion": once other possible causes have been ruled out, a diagnosis of IBS can be made. Although conventional tests usually fail to reveal any obvious physical abnormalities, internal examination using colonoscopy often reveals a normal looking intestine but with an abnormally high level of activity. So if there are no obvious physical abnormalities, what could be causing this extremely common problem?

To answer this problem, we need to go to the work of Dr. William Rea who has treated over 20,000 patients in his Dallas hospital, the Environmental Health Center, which specializes in the diagnosis and treatment of environmental diseases. What he has discovered is that IBS appears to be particularly influenced by environmental triggers, such as toxic chemicals, and a range of allergens, such as pollen and certain foods. The good news is that symptoms can often be eliminated by removing these triggers and lowering the total body's chemical-pollutant load.

HOW CHEMICALS AFFECT IBS

The problem appears to lie in the makeup of our gastrointestinal system and its extreme vulnerability to the harmful effects of chemicals. It seems that chemicals can totally disrupt the smooth functioning of virtually every aspect of bowel activity. The combination of chemicals that the intestines are exposed to from the diet, together with the on-going background exposure that all the body organs get from the ex-isting body burden of chemicals, means that our intestines tend to be the body parts exposed to the highest level of chemicals.

But rather than listing all the chemicals involved, it is more helpful to understand how our digestive system works and then the ways in which chemicals can interfere. This will make it easier to understand how chemicals can produce the wide range of symptoms, such as ex-cess gas, bloating, cramps, diarrhea, constipation, and excess mucus production, commonly experienced by IBS sufferers.

The layer of muscle in the bowel wall controls the diameter of the stool. When the muscle in the wall contracts, the diameter of the wall narrows and the bowel goes into spasm. When the muscle relaxes, its diameter increases and the bowel becomes dilated. Its degree of con-traction is regulated by a number of different hormones, nerves, min-eral levels, and overall body pH. Toxic chemicals can damage all these controlling factors.

Chemicals can also alter the rate and extent of bowel muscle contrac-tion, prompting prolonged periods of spasm or relaxation—a possible cause of the previously mentioned increased activity of the intestines commonly seen in IBS sufferers. This muscle spasm or dilatation could also lead to symptoms of bloating, diarrhea, and constipation. Another way in which chemicals produce symptoms of IBS is by increasing or decreasing the levels of mucus secretion. Chemical damage done to the balance of intestinal bacteria or microflora results in excess wind. The range of symptoms experienced depends upon which part of the gut is affected, as well as the particular damage done.

Toxic chemicals induce a range of symptoms in those who suffer from IBS. But the damage caused by chemicals is usually invisible on conventional tests, because they are not looking for it, which could ex-plain why these tests tend not to be able to find a physical cause for a patient's symptoms.

And while chemical exposure is usually not the only factor behind IBS, the number of people who appear to be particularly sensitive to the effects of chemicals is actually greater than may initially be imagined. In a study of normal and "healthy" older people, the majority (57 percent) reported that smelling one or more toxic chemicals (pesticides, automobile exhaust, paint, new carpet, perfume) brought on symptoms of IBS. Interestingly, the higher the number of chemicals people were affected by, the more likely they were to report symptoms of irritable bowel syndrome. As chemicals are known to induce symptoms of IBS, any program designed to ease these symptoms should include an element of both chemical avoidance and detox.

Restoring Digestive Health

The good news is that if the general detox principles described in this book are used to lower the level of toxins in food, as well as the overall body burden of chemicals, this could help prevent as well as ease the symptoms of many chemically linked digestive system diseases. I now know many people who, just by going on my detox program, have been cured of their IBS.

While it might not totally cure IBD or some food intolerances, adding detoxing to your health-care program is a sensible option that will lower the level of chronic inflammation, while calming down a supersensitive digestive system and preventing disease flare-ups.

Since most people get their biggest load of chemicals from food, eating less contaminated foods will not only dramatically cut the level of chemicals in your digestive system, but in your whole body as well. By paying attention to reducing our digestive system's exposure to chemicals, we find that energy levels improve, the skin becomes clearer, body odors are reduced, and the immune system is strengthened.

SUPPLEMENTS

Nutritional therapy is not only essential in enabling the detox process and lowering the body's existing chemical load, it is particularly important in people with digestive system disorders as they are generally more prone to nutritional deficiencies. This is because they are less able to absorb nutrients due to an increased level of inflammation, and also because cutting major food groups out of the diet, necessary for those with marked allergies, can further increase the chance of nutrient deficiencies.

The program suggested in this book is ideal for most people with mild to moderate disease. However, due to the extreme levels of nutrient deficiencies commonly found in people with severe inflammatory bowel disease, individual supplementation programs based on testing of nutrient levels might be more appropriate. This is because these people might initially need intravenous nutrition.

In addition, MSM-sulfur, and to some degree the sulfur-containing amino acid supplements as listed in the supplement program in chapter 2, are not essential for people with inflammatory bowel diseases, who could potentially have an adverse reaction to compounds containing sulfur. Due to a malfunctioning detoxification system, some people with inflammatory bowel disease may experience particular difficulties in processing this compound.

All of the nutrients suggested in the general detox program should be beneficial, but magnesium is particularly useful as it can help relax bowel muscle spasms caused by chemically induced mineral imbalances and suppress immune system overactivity. Zinc helps by reducing the degree of bowel inflammation and reducing the symptoms of food intolerances.

Other nutrients of value are the antioxidants, such as vitamins C and E and selenium, as they appear to reduce the chemically induced immune system damage that is so commonly found in people with food intolerances. Vitamin B_6 is good for strengthening the immune system, while omega-3 oils suppress bowel inflammation.

If food intolerances continue for any period of time, or if milk products are cut from the diet, the levels of vitamins B_2 (riboflavin), B_3 (niacin), D, iron, and calcium can get very low, consequently any multivitamin and mineral supplement taken needs to contain adequate levels of these nutrients. Probiotics can also improve the bacterial balance of the bowel, making it less inflamed.

DIET

It is also important to discover and avoid the foods that your body has difficulty tolerating. If the problem is thought to arise from contact with cow's milk, then this should be eliminated from the diet; if it is gluten, then only gluten-free foods should be eaten. However, due to the real difficulty in determining which food is causing the problem, I would strongly recommend seeking the help of a nutrition or environmental health specialist not only in determining what the particular trigger is but also in managing the food allergy or intolerance.

One of the substances particularly effective in removing persistent chemicals from the digestive system is soluble fiber, such as that found in oatmeal, beans, apples, oranges, pectin, and psyllium seed. Soluble fiber also helps rebalance the microflora of the digestive system, since it acts as a food source for them. However, since psyllium can occasionally trigger allergic reactions (mainly in people who manufacture it naturally), it could in some cases be better, particularly if there is a suspicion of allergy to this substance, to use a soluble fiber that is hypoallergenic, such as pectin. Although insoluble fiber, or roughage, can help speed up the time that waste products spend in the body, thereby reducing the chances of chemicals being reabsorbed, care should also be taken to avoid wheat bran as this insoluble fiber could irritate the digestion further, particularly in those who are sensitive to wheat.

Other things that can help lower one's stress levels include learning to relax, taking up yoga, or going for long walks. Avoiding coffee, alcohol, and spices may also ease symptoms.

CHAPTER 8

Hormonal Imbalances

THE ESCALATING NUMBER OF PEOPLE developing hormone-related health problems, such as diabetes, thyroid disease, and infertility, indicates that there is something about modern-day life that appears to be playing havoc with our hormones. Scientists have now tracked the problem down to the myriad of chemicals in our environment and foods. It seems clear that many of the most common chemicals in our environment are capable of causing hormonal havoc.

Indeed, there is growing evidence that the levels at which chemicals can affect our hormones are the levels that we are now being exposed to. What's more, the levels currently found in our bodies are already thousands of times higher than the natural hormones they appear to mimic. So despite being much less potent than natural hormones, we know for a fact that many chemicals are already present in our bodies at levels that are affecting our hormones and damaging our health. To understand the potential health-damaging consequences of these hormone-disrupting substances, it helps to understand what hormones are, how they work, and what they do.

Our hormones are natural chemical molecules that act as internal messengers. They are produced in glandular tissue, and when released they carry information and instructions around the body, enabling one part to communicate with another. Although only minuscule amounts of hormones are produced, they control virtually all the body's functions—such as growth, reproduction, metabolism, and weight. Levels of these hormones are themselves controlled by a complex regulatory system that involves a degree of feedback control from the brain. The flexibility of the existing system is what has allowed humans to be so successful in adapting to a wide range of situations and environments. But this same flexibility appears to have opened it up to attack, as a blockage of one part can have serious repercussions for the smooth running of the rest.

Unfortunately for us, modern chemicals are able to not only damage one part of the hormonal system, but they possess an ability to interfere with the entire system. Not one of our major hormones is left untouched, as sex hormones, thyroid hormones, insulin, growth hormone, catecholamines (fight and flight hormones, which also control weight), and steroids, are all highly vulnerable to toxic-chemical damage.

The chemicals that affect our hormones include all the usual suspects, such as toxic metals, pesticides (every one I have ever studied disrupts the functioning of at least one major type of hormone), solvents, plasticizers, and halogen-containing substances such as chlorine, fluorine, and bromine. They can cause this damage because:

➤ Hormone-producing tissues (glands) are a particular target for blood-borne chemicals, due to their excellent blood supply.

➤ Hormone-producing tissues usually contain a higher proportion of fat, so they tend to accumulate more persistent fat-soluble toxins. Therefore these highly important and sensitive tissues often end up being some of the most polluted parts of our bodies.

➤ Chemicals can obstruct the creation of hormones.

➤ Chemicals can also impair the release of hormones from the glands.

➤ Many chemicals can mimic the action of natural hormones, and unlike natural chemicals that can be effectively switched off, there is no such mechanism present for the artificial hormone mimics.

➤ Chemicals can physically prevent natural hormones from working by coming between them and the tissue they need to stimulate.

➤ Chemicals damage the normal circadian rhythm of hormone
release, knocking millions of subsequent reactions out of sync.

➤ Toxins can dramatically change the rate at which hormones are
removed from the body. For instance, they can dramatically
increase the rate at which hormones are excreted, resulting in
lowered hormone levels.

The net result of all these effects is to seriously disrupt the way the entire body works, thus putting all the health systems under undue stress
and making them more disease prone.

Diabetes

Diabetes is one of the most serious diseases in the world, not only
because of the way it forces us to completely change the way we live or
the significant damage it, as a progressive disease, can cause to our
bodies, but because the number of people now getting it has gone
through the roof. Currently some 7 million Americans have type II diabetes. It gets worse: the World Health Organization has predicted that
between 1997 and 2035, the number of diabetics will double from 143
million to about 300 million.

The predicted dramatic escalation of diabetes within this short time
frame implies that this condition is strongly linked to new environmental factors such as chemicals. Indeed, some scientists now hold
these environmental factors responsible for up to 50 percent of the current cases. This powerful environmental connection can be clearly seen
when people move from an area with a relatively low risk of diabetes to
a high-risk area, as their risk of becoming diabetic climbs. To understand how chemicals can trigger diabetes, we first need to know what
diabetes is.

Diabetes is a serious hormonal and metabolic disorder caused by
the body's inability to deal with carbohydrates and sugars, resulting in

an abnormally high level of blood sugar. This is caused by either a total lack of insulin—insulin being a hormone that encourages the storage of sugars in the body after eating a meal—known as type I diabetes (formerly known as insulin-dependent diabetes), or a reduced ability of the body to respond to insulin, known as type II diabetes (formerly named non-insulin-dependent diabetes). One of the main problems diabetics face are the long-term serious health complications associated with this condition, such as diabetic retinopathy, kidney failure, heart disease, and diabetic neuropathy.

How Chemicals Can Trigger Diabetes

Many chemicals are not only able to trigger diabetes in those with an inherited tendency to the disease, they can also induce diabetes in those with no family history. Several synthetic chemicals are even used to trigger diabetes in animals to create models of the disease. This powerful diabetogenic ability appears to stem from an ability to damage the hormone systems that control sugar metabolism by altering levels of hormones that are vital to carbohydrate metabolism, such as insulin, by directly targeting and destroying insulin-producing cells and by interfering with a large number of other carbohydrate-controlling mechanisms.

The reason that we are seeing the number of people with diabetes rise could be a direct result of our ever-increasing exposure to these diabetogenic substances.

Evidence for a significant change in the main underlying causes of diabetes is reflected in a change in the fundamental nature and pattern of the disease. For example, not only have steep rises been documented in the number of children affected by type I diabetes, but the age at which children develop the disease has dramatically fallen. This is even more marked in the case of type II diabetes, a disease previously only known to affect adults that is now affecting more and more children.

The rise in early-onset diabetes could be because chemicals tend to be far more toxic and cause greater damage to the bodies of developing babies than to adults. The increasing body burden of chemicals in mothers' bodies could explain why diabetes is affecting people at an ever-younger age. It would also explain why children of older mothers (with their higher body burdens of chemicals) and first-born children (who tend to get the biggest load of chemicals from their mothers) have an even higher risk of developing diabetes.

Many chemicals appear to be linked to diabetes, but one of the most important groups of diabetogenic chemicals out there are the organo-chlorine pesticides and environmental contaminants. The higher the level of these common contaminants in the body, the greater the risk of developing diabetes. Organochlorines appear to be so strongly linked to this disease because of their powerful ability to interfere with normal

Chemicals That Trigger and Exacerbate Diabetes

Alcohol

Cigarette smoke

Environmental pollutants (dioxin, PCBs)

Food contaminants (nitrate from artificial fertilizers, inorganic bromide)

Organochlorine pesticides (such as DDT)

Pesticides (herbicides, organophosphates, carbamates)

Pharmaceutical drugs (antibiotics such as penicillin, cephalo-sporin, and erythromycin; blood pressure medications; nifedip-ine; diuretics such as frusemide and chlorthiazide; sedatives such as benzodiazepine, tranquilizers, and barbiturates; and painkillers such as paracetamol)

Preservatives

Solvents (e.g., benzene)

Toxic metals (arsenic, mercury, lead)

carbohydrate metabolism. The good news is that lowering the body levels of these chemicals can reverse much of this damage. However, since organochlorines are stored in body fat, any form of rapid weight loss results in the mobilization of large amounts of these stored toxins into the bloodstream, where they are transported to vital body organs and cause even greater damage. If not anticipated and properly prepared for (by taking nutritional supplements and soluble fiber as described in this program), the subsequent damage could potentially double the long-term risk of developing diabetes.

People working with other types of pesticides, such as herbicides and insecticides, also have a higher risk of developing diabetes. As well as triggering hormonal damage, these chemicals can also cause dramatic swings in blood sugar levels. In fact, this diabetogenic nature of pesticides can be so powerful that one type of pesticide is used to induce diabetes in animals to create a model of the disease for research purposes. Diabetic animal models are also created by exposing animals to another form of artificial chemical in the form of an antibiotic known as streptozotocin. This chemical triggers the disease by poisoning insulin-producing cells.

Antibiotics are not the only synthetic medicines that possess powerful diabetic-inducing actions, as a large number of pharmaceutical drugs are known for this quality. This group covers a wide range of different drugs used as antibiotics, to treat high blood pressure (a recent UK government warning revealed that the common combination of beta-blockers and thiazide diuretic treatment for raised blood pressure results in a 20-percent-higher risk of developing diabetes than other treatments), as diuretics and sedatives, and for pain relief.

The list of chemicals linked to diabetes extends to cover many other groups such as the toxic metals. These appear to trigger diabetes by increasing levels of tissue-damaging free radicals. The higher the level of these toxic metals in the body, the greater the apparent diabetic risk. Higher exposure to chemicals from common water contaminants, such as the solvent benzene, and food contaminants, such as inorganic bromide, and nitrates from artificial fertilizers and preservatives are also linked to an increased risk of diabetes.

Thyroid Disease

If you are feeling tired all the time, have lost your vital spark, and seem to have forgotten what it is like to feel normal, it may not be due to your age—you could be one of the millions of people whose thyroid hormone is not working properly. Some specialists estimate that approximately one in five people over fifty-five is now affected, though only one in one hundred people are diagnosed with an underactive thyroid. Thus, the vast majority of sufferers are potentially missing out on a wealth of restorative treatment and a far better quality of life.

But it is not just the number of people with underactive thyroids on the increase, other common forms of thyroid disease are also becoming much more common. These include thyroid cancer, which in Australia has increased thirtyfold in the space of four decades, and overactive thyroids, which in some populations have increased more than three times over the last ten years.

To understand why thyroid diseases are on the increase, we need to know a bit more about how the thyroid works. The thyroid gland is situated in the neck and produces two types of thyroid hormones: T3 (triiodothyronine) and T4 (L-tetraiodothyronine). These hormones are periodically released into the blood, where most of them bind onto specially created proteins and are carried around the body to wherever they are needed. Thyroid hormones are essential because they control the metabolic rate (power metabolism, burn fat, and stimulate carbohydrate utilization); stimulate growth; facilitate weight control; allow normal development of the brain in babies; are essential hormones in reproduction; and allow the heart and cardiovascular system to work properly.

Controlling the thyroid gland is a complex business; proper functioning relies on many factors such as nerve signals from the brain, adequate levels of nutrition, and feedback from existing levels of thyroid hormones in the body. When things go wrong, the end result is usually one of two conditions: hypothyroidism (abnormally low levels of thyroid hormones, which cause symptoms of weakness, fatigue, muscle and joint ache, and weight gain) and hyperthyroidism (too many thyroid hormones, which cause symptoms of increased nervousness; weight loss; increased sweating, fatigue, and weakness; and prominent eyes). However, with the number of people developing thyroid cancer rising, we need to discover what is poisoning our thyroid glands.

CHEMICALS AND THYROID DISEASE

There is compelling evidence linking thyroid disease with the increased chemicalization of our environment. And it's not just those working with chemicals who are at risk. Current levels of environmental pollution have resulted in us all being in the firing line. Those who actually go on to develop thyroid diseases probably do so from a combination of the following factors: an increased genetic susceptibility to thyroid disease; previous exposure to thyroid-damaging toxins; chemical exposure at a young age (the earlier the exposure, the greater the damage); and history of inadequate nutrition (those with a poor diet are more at risk from chemical damage).

When I was researching my previous book on how chemicals affect our weight, I examined the effect on the thyroid gland by each of the major types of chemicals we are now exposed to. I was shocked to find that the majority of these chemicals have some sort of thyroid-damaging potential. Not only do different chemicals possess the ability to increase or decrease the level of thyroid hormone in the body, some chemicals can induce both conditions under differing circumstances, and other synthetic chemicals are known to increase the risk of thyroid cancer.

The herbicides, insecticides, and fungicides commonly found in our foods contain some of the most powerful thyroid-hormone suppressors known. Some, like the carbamates, are actually used for this very purpose in animals, to make them put on weight faster, and in humans, as common medications to suppress an overactive thyroid. The extensive usage of pesticides on our fields means that in many agricultural regions, these thyroid-damaging chemicals are also seeping into our water supply.

There is also a powerful link between the levels of environmental pollutants, such as HCB, PCBs, and dioxin, in our bodies and the level

Chemicals Known to Damage the Thyroid Gland

Conventional therapeutic drugs

Environmental pollutants (such as PCBs, PBBs, dioxin)

Food additives and preservatives

Halogens (such as chlorine, bromide, and fluoride)

Meat contaminants (from animal growth promoters and veterinary medicines)

Pesticides (such as DDT, lindane, HCB, organophosphates, and carbamates)

Plastics

Solvents

Synthetic rubber

Toxic metals (such as mercury)

of our thyroid hormone. In many cases, the more polluted the body is, the lower the level of thyroid hormones in the blood.

Toxic metals such as mercury can damage thyroid functioning by increasing the risk of autoimmune thyroid disease and by increasing the risk of developing thyroid cancer. Synthetic compounds such as plastics and synthetic rubber also appear to add to the problem. For instance, workers engaged in the production of synthetic rubber revealed a high (35 percent) prevalence of thyroid disease. Indeed, the longer the time spent working with these chemicals, the lower the levels of thyroid hormones detected in the blood. Phthalates, the chemicals that make plastics flexible, and one of the most common types of environmental pollutants, also appear to possess powerful antithyroid attributes.

Fertility Problems

Becoming pregnant and managing to carry a child to term appears to be a growing problem in our modern world. A surprising 8 to 12 percent of couples worldwide are thought to be infertile, and many top scientists predict that this number is set to increase still further.

The heartache that this problem causes is incalculable since few problems are as distressing as an inability to conceive. Not only can the basic instinct to have a child be very powerful, in many countries being childless is viewed as socially unacceptable. The burning need for children can result in vast sums of money being spent on high-tech fertility techniques, which not only are very expensive but also have very significant health risks attached.

After many years working in the field of environmental medicine, what really surprises me is not that the infertility rate is so high, but that so many healthy babies are still being born at all. Indeed, the discovery that current levels of pollution were causing infertility and reproductive problems in our wildlife is what brought me to this field in the first place.

How Chemicals Damage Fertility Levels

While many of the causes of infertility have been documented and known about for years, growing attention is now being directed to the effects that toxic chemicals have on our fertility. Chemicals are well-known for having the ability to seriously damage every aspect of our fertility. Chemically induced changes in sex hormone levels will damage sexual behavior, "feminize" boys and "masculinize" girls, as well as directly poison sperm and eggs, making them less fertile and more likely to abort or miscarry if they do get fertilized.

It may be no coincidence that since the 1950s, synthetic chemical production has increased fivefold, while the average sperm count has dropped by more than half. In light of the known detrimental effect chemicals have on sperm production, this dramatic fall in sperm count comes as little surprise.

Early warning signs about the damage artificial chemicals can cause to human reproduction first emerged a couple of decades ago when a U.S. fertility clinic started to notice that they were seeing an increasing number of people who worked in a factory that manufactured pesticides. Further observations revealed that the longer the duration of pesticide exposure, the lower the sperm count dropped: the longer men were exposed to this pesticide, the fewer sperm they had. Worse still, after a couple of years of working with this particular pesticide, sperm production totally and irreversibly ceased in many, leaving them irreversibly infertile. Although this particular pesticide (1,2-dibromo-3-chloropropane [DBCP]) was banned in the United States, it is still being used in other countries, and is continuing to devastate the fertility and the lives of the people who are exposed to it.

Despite the apparent slump in our fertility levels, the situation can potentially be reversed by making a deliberate effort to lower our exposure to chemical toxins. This was shown in a group of organic farmers who ate a higher proportion of organic foods than did the general population and were found to have almost double the sperm count.

In order to reverse this situation, we first need to know which chemicals do the most damage to fertility, so we can devise ways of avoiding them or minimizing their toxicity. By understanding this problem, we are one step away from finding significant and effective ways of dealing with it.

Other studies have looked at the level of pesticides in those women undergoing in vitro fertilization (IVF) and have discovered that the higher the level of toxins detected in body fluids, particularly of the persistent pesticides and environmental pollutants known as organochlorines, the lower the chances of successful fertilization. IVF rates are also significantly lower if the male partner has had previous exposure to pesticides. As pesticides are designed to kill all forms of life and to suppress reproduction in unwanted bugs and animals, these antifertility effects should come as little surprise.

Increased exposure to toxic metals such as mercury and lead is also linked to infertility. Unfortunately, studies show that the levels that affect fertility appear to be those at which we are currently exposed. For

Chemicals Known to Reduce Fertility and Increase Instance of Miscarriage

Bromine (a food contaminant)

Cigarette smoke

Environmental pollutants (such as PCBs and dioxin)

Organochlorine pesticides (such as DDT)

Pesticides (the vast majority of them)

Plastics

Solvents

Substances containing chlorine (e.g., the disinfectant in tap water)

instance, couples who eat greater amounts of seafood tend to have higher body levels of mercury, and the higher the level of mercury, the greater the infertility. Higher body levels of mercury are also found in people with a large number of amalgam (mercury-containing) fillings. Fortunately, it seems that if levels of toxic metals are lowered using specially targeted supplements (as are found in this program) then the chance of conception can be greatly improved.

Research into chlorine by-product levels in tap water, as a consequence of water chlorination, found that chlorine by-products in water may harm the developing fetuses, increasing the risk of miscarriage and birth defects.

How to Improve Hormonal Health

To obtain optimal hormonal health it is vital to start tackling the buildup of existing chemicals in the body by reducing the daily exposure to toxins, in combination with tackling the existing body burdens. This can result in better diabetes control, and occasionally, in type II diabetes, it has resulted in a cure. It can also help lower the odds of getting thyroid cancer and help optimize thyroid hormone functioning.

For those with fertility problems, it appears clear that to optimize your chances of becoming pregnant and having a healthy baby, it would be sensible to reduce the regular exposure to chemicals as well as the existing body burden in both prospective parents. While reducing chemicals is sensible at any time and particularly during pregnancy, deliberate attempts to lower existing body burdens of chemicals that involve fasting or severe food restriction should be done a couple of months before any attempts to become pregnant have been made because active detoxification can mobilize toxins and potentially affect the developing fetus.

Supplements

Proper nutrition also plays a vital role in optimizing hormonal health. This is particularly obvious when you discover that people who have nutrient deficiencies are at greater risk of developing hormonal imbalances. Indeed, certain hormonal diseases themselves increase the demand for nutrients; for example, people with overactive thyroid glands tend to need a higher level of antioxidants.

Good nutrition also strengthens the body's ability to protect itself against the damage done by toxins, by soaking up excess free radicals and boosting the body's ability to rid itself of chemicals. The supplement plan suggested in chapter 2 provides a good general level of nutrition that should be of benefit to all those with existing hormonal imbalances. It will also help to strengthen the hormonal system and, in so doing, reduce the chance of future disease.

For those wanting to improve fertility, optimal nutrition for *both* partners is vital for not only increasing the chances of becoming pregnant but also in reducing the risk of miscarriage and having a healthy child. If actively trying for a baby, it is wise for the woman to take supplements specifically designed for pregnancy as the levels of certain nutrients need to be limited, such as restricting vitamin A to a maximum of 10,000 IU a day. As it takes three months for sperm to develop and one month for the egg or ovum, good nutrition during this time will really boost the odds for becoming pregnant and having fewer complications throughout.

People with existing thyroid disease may find that, despite a generally increased need for nutrients, certain types of supplements may disagree with them. So it may be better to start off by taking one type of supplement, then introducing a new one every few days. This makes it easier to isolate and discontinue any potentially problematic supplements.

DIET

Other general ways in which to boost hormonal health include cutting down on the levels of toxins consumed by following the Seven-Day Desludge Diet; reducing the levels of stimulants in your diet, such as coffee, cigarettes, and tea; and cutting down on refined sugar. In addition to diet, increase the amount of regular exercise you take. Get at least thirty minutes of exercise, three times a week.

CHAPTER 9

Cardiovascular Diseases

A STAGGERING ONE OUT OF every two people dies from heart disease, yet just over one hundred years ago, heart attacks were virtually unheard of. This extraordinary emergence of a disease over what is at most a couple of generations reflects the dramatic changes in the environment, diet, and lifestyles that have taken place over this time.

The characteristics of those developing heart attacks and many other heart conditions continues to change and evolve, possibly due to the changing incidence of risk factors in the population such as smoking, high cholesterol, high blood pressure, obesity, diabetes, and poor nutrition.

But despite in-depth research on a few well-known risk factors, there appears to be a gaping hole in our knowledge base when it comes to looking at the effect many modern toxic chemicals have on heart disease, which is surprising in light of their well-known toxicities and their ever-growing presence in our lives.

If you consider that the cardiovascular system is controlled by hormones and nerves and made up of different kinds of muscle tissue in the heart and the blood vessels, all of which are known to be vulnerable to chemical damage, it stands to reason that these systems would be affected in some way. Yet despite a well-known link between chemicals and cardiovascular damage, this particular form of toxicity is currently very much underrated and not well known by either the general physician or layperson.

This has great significance for the individual who has or is developing heart problems, as he or she could be failing to address the source of the problem. Since cardiovascular disease is now so common, any additional knowledge on a potentially reversible problem, such as chemical damage, could make all the difference between life and death for millions of people worldwide.

Numerous studies show that certain groups of people who are exposed to higher levels of particular chemicals in different aspects of their working or ordinary lives, such as cleaners or industrial workers, are at a higher risk of developing cardiovascular diseases. The type of chemical a person works with tends to determine the type of disease they will get. Chemicals implicated here include all the usual suspects, such as pesticides, environmental pollutants, toxic metals, solvents, plastics, chlorine, and fluoride.

For instance, high blood pressure appears to be most strongly connected to an increased exposure to toxic metals, whereas higher blood fat (lipids), high cholesterol levels, and diabetes, all tend to have powerful associations with increased levels of organochlorine pesticides and environmental pollutants. So while it is a good idea to reduce your intake of all toxic chemicals, if you have a particular disease, target the chemicals that are known to be linked to it.

High Cholesterol

For the last few decades, many millions of people have been waging a war against higher levels of cholesterol. The strong link between increased levels of cholesterol and a higher risk of heart disease has resulted in vast sums of money being spent on testing for and treating higher levels of cholesterol as a way of preventing heart disease. However, this "treatment" can cause health problems due to the many known, and frequently extreme, toxicities of the drugs known collectively as statins.

For many people, the first advice in tackling high cholesterol is to cut down on dietary cholesterol, but this alone often makes very little impact on overall body levels. However, when I was researching my first book, *The Body Restoration Plan,* I looked at the effect toxic chemicals had on cholesterol levels. The more studies I read, the more apparent it became that the major types of toxic chemicals now found in our bodies can significantly increase blood levels of cholesterol.

Despite the effective demonization of the fat or lipid known as cholesterol in our current society, the truth is that we all need a certain amount of it in our bodies, otherwise we would most certainly die, as cholesterol helps create and maintain the shape and structure of all our cells. Cholesterol is also an essential precursor of many vital hormones, such as male and female sex hormones and steroids, as well as being a precursor of vitamin D. This is why certain drugs that simply prevent cholesterol from being made, such as the statins, have other health-damaging effects in that they lead to subnormal production of hormones and other useful substances made from cholesterol. Side effects linked to the use of these substances include a lowered sex drive, less energy, weight gain, dizziness, painful muscle cramps (they nearly crippled my mother in the few days she took them), cancer, and the list goes on and on. One source I saw listed over one hundred potential side effects. And these drugs are meant to "prevent" us from getting ill?

There are two main sources of cholesterol, LDL (or low-density lipoprotein), commonly known as the bad cholesterol because it is more likely to be deposited in the artery wall as a fatty atheromatous plaque, and HDL (or high-density lipoprotein), which is the good cholesterol, as it can declog arteries of deposited cholesterol thereby cleansing them.

Cholesterols are used to help transport dietary fats (alternatively known as lipids such as triglycerides) around the body from the digestive system and into the bloodstream to the places they need to go. While everyone has different levels of cholesterol, the key to health is a balanced ratio of HDL and LDL in the body. The ideal ratio is one part HDL to three parts total cholesterol. The higher a person's HDL cholesterol compared to the LDL cholesterol, the lower the risk from heart disease. High levels of dietary fats or triglycerides are also linked to heart disease.

Chemicals can not only increase cholesterol levels, but also tend to simultaneously worsen the balance of good to bad cholesterol by interfering with and blocking the conversion of cholesterol into useful substances, such as hormones. Consequently, the levels of cholesterol build up while the levels of cholesterol-based hormones and other useful cholesterol-based substances decreases. Some of these chemicals can also increase the level of triglycerides.

The chemicals most strongly associated with this cholesterol-increasing effect appear to be the organochlorine pesticides and pollutants, such as DDT, lindane, PCBs, and dioxin. It seems that the higher the body levels of these highly persistent and exceedingly common body contaminants, the higher the level of cholesterol and triglycerides in the blood. Not only is this cholesterol-increasing effect found in people who work with these chemicals, but also in people who do not work with pesticides and are merely exposed to higher levels of these toxins from their environment and diet.

Chemicals Associated with High Cholesterol

Environmental pollutants (dioxin, PCBs)

Halogens (chlorine)

Medical drugs (such as oral contraceptives, thiazide diuretics, beta-blockers, calcium channel blockers, and corticosteroids)

Pesticides (organochlorines, organophosphates, carbamates)

Solvents (trichloroethylene and alcohol)

Toxic metals (lead, mercury, copper, cadmium)

Many commonly used pesticides, such as the insecticide known as organophosphate, also appear to increase the cholesterol levels by blocking the pathway by which cholesterol is converted into useful substances, such as hormones.

Toxic metal exposure is also strongly linked to higher cholesterol levels. For instance, metal workers exposed to higher levels of lead have been found to have higher levels of cholesterol. Workers exposed to copper and cadmium also have abnormally high levels of blood fats. But it's not just metal workers at risk, as people who are exposed to higher levels of mercury from their diet (for example from seafood) and from other sources such as amalgam fillings, have also been found to have higher levels of bad cholesterol and lower levels of good cholesterol.

Even those who drink chlorinated water appear to be at risk. A study in Wisconsin found that those living in communities that chlorinated their water had higher levels of blood cholesterol than people in communities that did not.

Solvents such as alcohol and the commonly used dry-cleaning agent and paint thinner trichloroethylene also appear to damage cholesterol metabolism. Since reducing your body's exposure to the above chemicals can result in lower cholesterol levels, it makes sense to do all you can to achieve this. As optimum nutrition plays a vital role in detoxing, and actively, significantly, and safely lowering cholesterol, this should be tackled simultaneously. Many people now use detoxing to safely lower blood cholesterol levels, including my mother.

Heart Disease

There appear to be two main ways in which toxic chemicals trigger heart problems. The first is mainly from an immediate poisoning action on the heart tissues, and the second arises from a longer term increase in risk factors related to exposure to toxic chemicals.

Starting off with the direct toxic actions chemicals have on heart tissue, the parts of the heart most sensitive to direct chemical damage are the nerves, the highly specialized heart cells (pacemakers) that control the rate at which the heart beats, and the coronary arteries. Poisoning to the nerves and pacemakers can trigger the spectrum of abnormal heart rhythms, or arrhythmias, while chemical damage to the coronary arteries can cause them to go into spasm, triggering angina or, if the reduction in blood flow is severe, even a heart attack.

Longer term heart damage can be caused from a higher background level of chemically triggered increases in factors predisposing to heart disease, such as diabetes, high cholesterol, or high blood pressure.

It did not take much research to discover that many chemicals appear to possess a powerful ability to damage the heart. It is not only people who work with chemicals who have toxicity levels high enough to cause damage: many of these substances are now so widespread that they are already present in the population in levels large enough to cause significant damage to the heart.

Starting with pesticides, direct exposure to some of the chemicals more commonly detected on our foods, such as organophosphates, carbamates, and organochlorine pesticides, greatly increases the

Chemicals Known to Damage the Heart

Air pollution (sulphur dioxide)

Environmental pollutants (dioxin, PCBs)

Halogens (chlorine, fluoride)

Pesticides (organophosphates, carbamates, organochlorines)

Plastics (vinyl chloride)

Solvents (motor exhaust)

Toxic metals (arsenic, lead, mercury)

chances of developing abnormal heart rhythms. This can be clearly seen in those who deliberately ingest these substances in order to harm themselves, or in those who are exposed to higher levels of these chemicals due to their lifestyles, diet, and environment. In addition, certain chemicals such as the organophosphates, found in fly sprays and many other products, can actually cause heart muscle to break down and dissolve.

Toxic metals, such as arsenic, lead, and mercury, are also strongly implicated in triggering heart disease, such as ischemic heart disease (narrowing of coronary arteries and decreased blood flow to the heart), heart failure, and abnormal heart rhythms. The higher the level of toxic metals in the body, the greater the risk of heart disease. For example, the 15 percent of the population with the highest levels of lead in their bodies (a group made up of both chemical workers and non–chemical workers) have a raised incidence of ischemic heart disease and abnormal heart rhythms, slow heart rates in this instance. Everyone is at risk from lead-induced heart damage, not just those working with lead.

Halogens, such as chlorine and fluoride, also trigger abnormal heart rhythms. In one study, two children accidentally exposed to cleaning fluid containing fluoride had potentially fatal arrhythmias. If you consider that fluoride is a well-known cardiac poison, this is hardly surprising. The simple action of drinking chlorinated drinking water during pregnancy is also known to increase the risk for congenital heart defects in the unborn baby.

Other heart toxic chemicals that ordinary citizens are exposed to in everyday life are the persistent environmental pollutants. This is revealed by the strong link between ischemic heart disease and the level of chemicals such as PCBs and dioxin in the body. Higher rates of ischemic heart disease are also found in populations with higher levels of air pollution from substances such as sulphur dioxide and solvents from motor exhaust. Indeed, a rise in air pollution levels will be followed by increased hospital admissions among people with heart problems from ischemic heart disease, such as heart attacks.

Hypertension

According to a study published in *Journal of the American Heart Association* in August 2004, the number of adults in the United States with high blood pressure increased 30 percent over the last decade (from 1988 to 2000). The study concluded that almost a third of U.S. adults appear to have hypertension. So what is hypertension and what could be causing this massive increase?

Hypertension is the medical term for raised blood pressure. Blood pressure is simply a measurement of the pressure at which the blood leaves the heart and enters the arteries. If it is too low (hypotension) then our body systems cut out and we end up fainting, because we are not getting enough nutrients to our vital organs, such as our brain. If the pressure is too high (hypertension), then this can cause another set of problems such as increasing the risk of strokes or heart disease.

Blood pressure tends to be raised if there is an obstruction in the flow of the blood, from, say, arteries blocked with fatty atheromatous plaques, or constricted blood vessels in spasm that have narrowed diameters. When arteries are constricted, the heart has to pump the blood a little harder to keep the flow going through the blood vessels at the same pace, thereby raising the blood pressure.

How Chemicals Can Trigger or Exacerbate Hypertension

There appear to be two main ways in which the following toxic chemicals are thought to cause high blood pressure. First, from their powerful ability to trigger contraction of the muscle layer in the blood vessel, making it go into spasm. Second, from their longer term actions in raising LDL cholesterol levels, increasing the size and number of atheromatous plaques formed, which then clog the insides of the blood vessels.

The greater the level of toxic metals detected in the body, the greater the overall blood pressure levels. Indeed, the link between certain toxic metals, such as lead, and high blood pressure has appeared to be so

Chemicals Associated with Hypertension

Environmental pollutants (dioxin, PCBs)

Halogens (chlorine and chlorine products, fluorine and its products)

Medical drugs (such as oral contraceptives, thiazide diuretics, beta-blockers, calcium channel blockers, and corticosteroids)

Pesticides (organochlorines, organophosphates, carbamates)

Plastics (vinyl chloride)

Solvents (trichloroethylene, benzene, zylene, and alcohol)

Toxic metals (lead, mercury, copper, cadmium)

VOCs (volatile organic compounds, e.g., carbon disulfide)

powerful that one academic article questions whether lead exposure could be the principal cause of essential hypertension, which is far and away the most common type of high blood pressure.

It is not just lead that appears to have this effect since people exposed to higher levels of mercury at their work, such as dentists, are at higher risk of developing hypertension. Children exposed to higher levels of mercury in the womb, from contaminated seafoods and from their mother's dental amalgam fillings, also have a greater chance of developing high blood pressure.

Currently used pesticides appear to possess both short-acting and longer-term blood-pressure-increasing effects. For instance, a raised blood pressure is found in those who have deliberately ingested commonly found pesticides, such as organophosphates and carbamates, in order to harm themselves. It is also found in those who have been exposed to pesticides over longer periods of time due to their work.

Unfortunately for all of us, one of the most persistent groups of environmental pollutants now found in all of our bodies is strongly linked to higher blood pressure. This is the organochlorines family, and includes the now banned pesticide DDT, the industrial pollutants, PCBs, and dioxin. The higher the levels of these substances in our bodies, the greater the blood pressure tends to be. Since most of these chemicals were banned decades ago, we get most of these chemicals through our food and via our polluted environment. Alcohol and other industrial solvents (benzene and xylene) found in paint, car exhaust, household cleaning solutions, and perfume can bring about high blood pressure.

Other chemicals linked to high blood pressure are chlorine (as in tap water), fluorocarbons, carbon disulfide, asbestos, ozone, and plastics. For example, factory workers exposed over a number of years to the plastic vinyl chloride are known to have a markedly higher chance of developing hypertension. The higher the level of the chemical in their bodies, the greater the risk of hypertension.

If you just think of all the places where you can now find plastics and all these other chemicals in our modern world, it is no wonder that more and more people are developing high blood pressure.

Stroke

Few things can be as frightening as being fine one minute and being struck down the next, without any warning, killed or suffering from a sudden loss of basic physical and mental skills. Yet this is the situation millions of people find themselves in every day after having a stroke. The nightmare does not end there for those who survive this disaster, as many of the survivors are left with extensive physical and mental problems. Strokes are the most prevalent cause of adult disability in the Western world.

Stroke is a nonspecific term for the wide-ranging symptoms, such as paralysis, speech difficulties, and loss of certain mental abilities, caused by brain tissue damage. In most cases (approximately 85 percent) of stroke, this brain damage follows a sudden cut in the blood supply to a part of the brain because of a blockage in the blood vessel supplying the brain tissue with nutrients. This type of stroke is called a cerebral infarction. The other main cause of stroke results from a bleed into the brain from a ruptured blood vessel. This is known as a cerebral hemorrhage. The type and extent of symptoms experienced by an individual depend on the part of the brain that has been affected and the extent to which the damage extends through the brain.

Cerebral infarctions are caused by diseased or severely narrowed blood vessels or a blood clot, both of which can effectively block the blood vessel supplying one part of the brain. Often the two are present together, as blood clots tend to form on diseased blood vessels. Cerebral hemorrhages tend to be caused when existing weaknesses in the brain's blood vessels are stressed to the point of rupturing. These weaknesses can be triggered by high blood pressure (hypertension, see page 190) or from existing blood vessel disease, such as atherosclerosis from high cholesterol levels.

STROKES—THE CHEMICAL CONNECTION

Chemicals are very strongly linked to strokes from their ability to trigger some of the major stroke risk factors such as excess weight, high blood pressure, stress, diabetes, high blood lipids (cholesterol), and thick blood (polycythemia). In addition to a long list of chemicals that include the usual ones of pesticides (organophosphates), organochlorines, toxic metals (e.g., arsenic, cadmium, lead, and mercury), cigarette smoke, and air pollutants, there are many medicinal drugs that can directly trigger strokes.

Many chemicals used in therapeutic medicines are the same or at least very similar to many of those used as pesticides. Consequently, you don't have to be deliberately taking a medication to be exposed to a stroke-inducing chemical, since many could be present in your foods as pesticide residues, exposing you without your knowledge or consent.

Despite the existing evidence, the link between stroke and chemicals is not widely known. So few of those trying to avoid a stroke will have been adequately informed about the importance of lowering their personal exposure to toxic chemicals. If you consider that strokes are

Drugs That Contain Chemicals Known to Contribute to Stroke

Blood-pressure-lowering drugs (such as nifedipine and beta-blockers)

Chemotherapy medications

Clot-thinning medications (subcutaneous heparin and anti-coagulant medication)

Hormones (such as those given during chemotherapy, the contraceptive pill, oral anticoagulant therapy, and anabolic steroids)

Migraine drugs

Nasal decongestives (excessive use of)

Recreational drugs (Ecstasy, cocaine, and methamphetamines)

the third most common cause of death in the U.S., the sheer numbers involved would suggest that this should be an extremely worthwhile consideration for many, particularly if they are considered to be at high risk.

For those that look, direct links between pesticides and stroke can be found. For instance, carbamates, chemicals commonly used as a pesticide, can not only trigger strokes but can also increase the degree of brain damage following a stroke. Exposure to organophosphates, also commonly used as chemical pesticides, can bring about symptoms almost identical to a stroke, and workers exposed to organochlorine pesticides over the long term are at a higher risk of developing a stroke. Lastly, there is a wealth of evidence that links a wide range of pesticides to many of the other major stroke risk factors, such as obesity, diabetes, and hypertension.

Toxic metals are also linked to stroke. For instance, a study investigating the long-term risks of arsenic exposure (from contaminated water and other environmental sources) reveals that the higher the exposure, the greater the risk of developing a stroke. Cigarette smoke, which also contains several toxic metals, such as cadmium, can also increase the stroke risk. As with pesticides, toxic metals can also play an important role in the development of many stroke risk factors, such as the important role played by lead and mercury in causing high blood pressure (see page 190).

Air pollutants such as sulphur dioxide and carbon monoxide also appear to increase the stroke risk. One South Korean study revealed that higher levels of air pollution caused an increase in the number of people getting strokes.

Strengthening Your Cardiovascular System

The detox and chemical avoidance program found in this book is ideal for all those who wish to prevent and minimize symptoms of the previously mentioned cardiovascular diseases. For many people these diseases can eventually be controlled by chemical avoidance and adequate nutrients alone. Considering the often extreme side effects that accompany most drugs used to treat high blood pressure and cholesterol, the program outlined in Part I has to be a better way.

SUPPLEMENTS

Good nutrition and supplementation is critical in not only helping the body rid itself of cardiovascular system–damaging toxins, but also essential in keeping the underlying structure of the cardiovascular system in good working order. People deficient in certain nutrients tend to be at a much higher risk of developing cardiovascular illnesses. For instance, low levels of magnesium (commonly known as the relaxing mineral) can cause blood vessel constriction and raised blood pressure, while magnesium supplementation causes muscle relaxation and a lowering of the blood pressure. In addition, lower blood levels of the vitamins B_6, B_{12}, and folic acid tend to result in higher levels of a protein known as homocysteine. Excessively high levels of this protein are linked to increased rates of heart disease and high blood pressure. Fortunately, supplementation with these nutrients reduces the levels of homocysteine back to normal, and also reduces the risk of heart disease.

Nutrients with antioxidant properties also appear to play an important role in preventing and treating many cardiovascular diseases such as stroke and high blood pressure. Other nutrients, such as minerals, amino acids/MSM-sulfur, and essential fatty acids, are also of great value in optimizing cardiovascular health.

DIET

Soluble fiber, like that found in oatmeal, apples, oranges, beans, psyllium seed husks, and pectin, is an extremely effective and nontoxic way to significantly lower blood cholesterol to safe levels as it physically binds to the cholesterol and carries it out of the body. As many of the body's most persistant chemicals tend to be carried in fatty cholesterol, removing cholesterol in this way is also a very effective way of simultaneously detoxing the body.

CHAPTER 10

Cancer

THE WORST PART OF BEING a doctor is telling someone that they have cancer. This unenviable task never got any easier for me with time, because for each and every one of the people affected the news always came as a hard, cruel blow. In a flash, people often fear the worst as they instantly remember the people they have known or loved who succumbed to this often-unforgiving disease. They act as their own witnesses to the fact that many conventional cancer therapies, in addition to being extremely toxic, often fail to provide a really effective cure. If they were effective, getting cancer would not be so feared.

Despite repeated fanfares heralding new cancer-treating agents, the fact of the matter is that more and more people are developing cancer. In America the number of people with this disease has escalated to epidemic proportions, now striking 1.3 million, and killing about 550,000 annually. Nearly one in two men and more than one in three women will now develop cancer in their lifetimes.

Cancer occurs when our bodies are exposed to a factor or combination of factors that damage normal cells and makes them start dividing uncontrollably. It reflects a failure of our bodies' natural anticancer-forming systems (largely made up by our immune system) to work properly in removing the constant supply of abnormal cells that our bodies regularly throw out.

Of all the different substances known to cause cancer—commonly referred to as carcinogens—chemicals appear to play a very prominent role. The list of known cancer-causing chemicals is extremely long and getting longer by the day. It includes a roll-call of the usual suspects, such as pesticides, environmental pollutants, toxic metals, solvents, plastics, fluoride, and many other types of man-made chemicals found in our everyday environment, and foods, such as the synthetic steroids and artificial growth hormones used to fatten up U.S. beef cattle and increase production of milk. Synthetic steroids and growth hormone have both been banned in Europe as carcinogens.

However, the real situation could be far worse than already suspected, as a U.S. governmental oversight agency revealed that in 1987, of the more than 50,000 chemicals in commercial use, only 284 had been tested on animals for their cancer-causing potential by the government in the preceding ten years. Of these, 144 (about half) had been shown to cause cancer in animals. So, somewhat incredibly, the vast majority of industrial chemicals now in use have never been tested for their carcinogenic properties. One can only speculate what the results would be if such tests were to be carried out. Therefore, the assumption that most of us make that if something is for sale, everything in it has already undergone a thorough battery of tests and been found totally safe, is no longer valid, if indeed it ever was.

Not only do chemicals trigger a wide range of adult and childhood cancers—the most common being prostate, breast, brain, immune system (lymphomas and leukemias), urinary tract, and liver—they can also stimulate cancer growth in general, making a wide range of existing cancers much more aggressive and enhance their ability to spread throughout the body.

This raises the question why, in the light of all this evidence, conventional cancer specialists are ignoring the carcinogenic role of chemicals. This failure to grasp the chance to lower our exposure and body burden of known cancer-causing agents is a serious omission and a missed opportunity. Who knows how many people could have been saved if these issues had been properly addressed. This indifference is all the more surprising in the light of a U.S. government–sponsored safety and health document, produced by the Civil Service Employees Association (CSEA) Occupational Safety and Health department. U.S. government scientists have now estimated that as many as 33 percent of all cancers are related to workplace exposures to carcinogens. Considering that chemicals make up the majority of these carcinogens, and that we are also exposed to these chemicals in our homes, the true extent to which chemicals are triggering cancer is likely to be much greater. With statistics like these, is it any wonder that so many people are getting cancer?

The good news about knowing what triggers and exacerbates cancer, is that perhaps for the first time you can start effectively fighting back. Not only will the nontoxic methods of detoxing, chemical avoidance, and nutritional support help lower your odds of getting cancer in the future, they can also significantly improve your body's own natural ability to attack and kill existing cancer cells, often with astonishing results.

Breast Cancer

With breast cancer now being the most common cause of cancer death in women worldwide, and the numbers of those getting cancer showing no signs of slowing down, we are facing a catastrophic global epidemic. Not only would finding a cause help prevent millions from getting this cancer in the future, but it would also potentially help the millions already affected.

Despite the known link between breast cancer and the genetic inheritance, the rapid explosion in numbers suggests that other factors, especially environmental factors, are at work here. This fits in with other observations like the fact that women migrating from a low-risk to a high-risk area eventually acquire the higher risk. Indeed, when one scientist, Professor William Rea, MD, founder of the Environmental Health Center in Dallas, tried to determine the extent to which environmental factors play a role in the current epidemic, he found that they figured in an astonishing 95 percent of cases. Not surprisingly, chemicals feature highly on this group of environmental factors.

Although the exact mechanisms for chemicals' role in promoting breast cancer are as yet unknown, one way could be via the ability to generally increase levels of cancer-inducing free radicals, while another could be by damaging DNA proteins. Another appears to be due to an ability, possessed by a large and diverse number of chemicals, to mimic the actions of female hormones. These substances are often referred to as xenoestrogens (*xeno,* "foreign" and *estrogen,* female hormone).

To appreciate why these xenoestrogens appear to be so important in breast cancer, it helps to have an overview of the strong relationship between the hormones these chemicals mimic, namely the estrogens, and breast cancer.

Chemicals That Can Cause Breast Cancer

Alcohols

Chemicals containing chlorine

Detergents

Organochlorines (DDT, lindane, dieldrin, PCBs)

Pesticides (organophosphates, synthetic pyrethroids)

Plastics (bisphenol A, chloride)

Solvents (chlorinated)

Synthetic estrogens used in hormone replacement and the contraceptive pill

Toxic metals (tributyltin, cadmium, antimony, barium, chromium, lithium, lead acetate)

ESTROGENS—THE JEKYLL-AND-HYDE EFFECT

Estrogens are one of the hormones that make women different from men and play a fundamental role in controlling all aspects of female fertility. So it's alarming to discover that our own natural estrogens have been classified as known human carcinogens. Nonetheless, this darker side goes some way toward explaining the increasingly numerous reports finding that estrogens in the contraceptive pill and hormone replacement therapy are a cause of breast cancer.

This cancer-provoking effect appears to arise from the natural ability of estrogens to switch on breast cell growth and turnover. Both natural and synthetic estrogens dock onto highly specialized receptor sites in breast tissue, which turns on the inbuilt switch for triggering cell division. Then, almost as soon as the cell is switched on, this mechanism is turned off, because the estrogen is grabbed by a highly specialized protein that binds to it tightly, preventing it from getting free and stimulating more tissue.

Excessive stimulation of these receptor sites from higher levels of either natural or synthetic estrogens is thought to be one of the main factors behind normal cells turning cancerous. It also is likely that these substances make existing cancer cells more aggressive.

Since estrogens can trigger breast cancer, it seems logical that chemicals that can mimic the actions of estrogens should also be able to trigger breast cancer. While the strength of the breast cell stimulation triggered by xenoestrogens is generally much weaker than that caused by natural hormones, their fat-loving nature in combination with the high percentage of fat tissue in breasts means that xenoestrogens are now present in breast tissue in levels hundreds of times greater than the hormones they mimic. In addition, our bodies also appear to lack the ability to remove many xenoestrogens from breast cells once they have docked on, due to their widely varying forms.

The upshot of this is that breast cells end up getting falsely stimulated twenty-four hours a day. A vast number of chemicals are now known to mimic the effect of natural estrogens from those found in pesticides and plasticizers to common foods and personal care products. Indeed, due to the major extent in which xenoestrogens have crept into virtually every aspect of our lives, our modern environment has been likened by scientists to "living in a sea of estrogens."

Chemical Xenoestrogens

While you may think that this ability of chemicals to mimic estrogens is largely accidental, in some instances this could not be further from the truth. Take, for example, the plastic known as bisphenol A. Its adaptability has made it into one of the most commonly used plastics today, and it can be found in a whole range of products, from the inside coating of food tins to dental fillings and milk bottles for babies. However, few realize that this plastic was first developed in the 1930s as a potential synthetic form of estrogen. A paper published in the British medical journal *Lancet* in 1936 revealed research to that effect. So, far from accidentally possessing estrogen-mimicking properties, it seems that this plastic was specifically created for that purpose.

Another chemical that turns compounds into xenoestrogens is the element chlorine. This chemical, used as a weaponized gas in the First World War, can now be found in an extremely large number of synthetic chemicals, many of which have been found to promote breast cancer. At the simplest level, those who drink chlorinated water are at a higher risk of developing breast cancer. It seems that chlorine reacts with some of the substances in the water to form trihalomethanes, compounds linked to breast cancer. This cancer-inducing effect has been demonstrated in a study performed on women drinking chlorinated tap water in Louisiana.

Other chlorine-containing chemicals known to cause breast cancer are the organochlorines. This notorious, highly toxic and persistent group of chemicals includes the pesticides DDT and lindane, as well as the environmental pollutants, such as PCBs and dioxin. Much of the research into chemicals and breast cancer includes studies that have found breast cancer patients to have higher levels of these chemicals in their breast tissue and blood.

Prostate Cancer

Prostate cancer is already extremely widespread. Indeed, it currently holds the dubious honor of being the most common malignancy found in American males and the fourth most common cancer in the world. The number of new cases of American men diagnosed with prostate cancer between 1983 and 1989 rose by a hefty 6.4 percent. In fact, the older a man is, the more likely he is to develop it. Hard statistics obtained from autopsies of men who have died from other causes reveal that a staggering 40 percent of men over the age of fifty have prostate cancer. The risk increases as the decades pass, so by the age of eighty, a colossal 70 percent of American men have it. For men in their nineties, it's a near certainty.

But if you are a man reading this, don't get too depressed, because despite the seemingly high figures of those affected by prostate cancer, the fact remains that up to 90 percent never develop symptoms or become ill with it.

Knowing what helps some people to suppress cancer is critical because this information could be used to treat people with the disease while helping to prevent others from getting it. Recent breakthroughs have helped us understand that whether you become a victim or conqueror of this disease is largely determined by how exposed you are to toxic chemicals and the level of chemical detoxing nutrients in your diet.

THE EFFECT OF ARTIFICIAL CHEMICALS ON PROSTATE CANCER

Prostate cancer is one of the many cancers known to be powerfully triggered by a large number of chemicals currently found in our environment, such as pesticides, pollutants, toxic metals, plastics, and solvents. The levels of chemicals needed to trigger prostate cancer are not only encountered in those working with these substances on a day-to-day basis but, judging by the number of men who have already got this disease, it seems that the chemicalization of our everyday lives has put virtually every single man on the danger list.

As well as triggering the onset of prostate cancer, many now believe that chemical toxins can act on already established cancers to accelerate their growth, converting previously harmless cancers into killer cancers.

Scientists from the Medical College of Wisconsin have noted that aggressive prostate-cancer cells appeared to be different in their genetic makeup from dormant cells, and that environmental pollutants, such as toxic metals (particularly cadmium), cigarette smoke, pesticides, and automotive emissions, could bring about this transformation, turning non-aggressive prostate-cancer cells into these killer cells. They also found that exposure to these toxic pollutants could trigger aggressive cells to attack and invade the surrounding tissue, thus spreading the cancer through the body more rapidly.

Immune System Cancers: Lymphoma and Leukemias

Over the last few decades, the number of people with immune system cancers, such as lymphomas and leukemias, has been steadily increasing. The situation was thrown into the spotlight when Jacqueline Kennedy Onassis developed an increasingly common form of cancer, known as non-Hodgkin's lymphoma (NHL). Suddenly people started to sit up and take notice.

The rise of this cancer has been pretty marked, with the number of people developing it over the last twenty years rising by a massive 80 percent, and showing no signs of slowing. Indeed, with every passing year, the number of people developing NHL increases by approximately 3 percent, making it one of the fastest growing cancers in the world. This upsurge in a once-rare tumor has resulted in it now being the fifth most common cancer in the United States. But before we look at why this particular form of cancer is skyrocketing, it helps to know a bit more about immune system cancers.

The main forms of immune system cancers are leukemia, Hodgkin's lymphoma, non-Hodgkin's lymphoma, and multiple myeloma. While all of them have increased in incidence over the years, none of these increases have been as dramatic as those of non-Hodgkin's lymphoma. Despite having different names and characteristics, all these cancers originate from the cells that make up our immune system (see chapter 5), mainly the lymphocytes or white blood cells.

White blood cells play an essential role in protecting the body from all the infections and foreign bodies that we are exposed to. They are largely created in lymph nodes, which are kidney bean–shaped nodules scattered throughout the body. White blood cells travel around the body in the blood and lymph vessels. Some white blood cells specialize in producing vast quantities of proteins known as antibodies; other cells are designed to destroy infections directly on contact. The type of cancer one gets, and therefore one's symptoms and ultimate prognosis, depends on which type of cell becomes cancerous.

For instance, multiple myeloma occurs when a mature antibody-producing cell becomes cancerous and starts churning out excessively large quantities of antibodies that build up in the body tissues and can be detected in large quantities in the blood. Leukemia occurs when certain types of white blood cells start being produced in large numbers and found in excessive quantities in the bloodstream. And lymphomas occur when immune cells in lymph nodes start multiplying uncontrollably, resulting in an abnormally large lymph node.

THE LINK BETWEEN CHEMICALS AND IMMUNE SYSTEM CANCERS

To discover what might be behind this increase in immune system cancers, look at the people developing them: a large number are found in certain occupations, many involving exposure to high levels of chemicals. Chemical exposure is therefore high on the list of possible triggers for immune system cancers.

A large number of chemicals appear to trigger immune system cancers. But it is not just work exposure that appears to predispose to these cancers, because any form of exposure in our lives, such as treating the house with pesticides, can result in a higher rate of cancer.

My husband lost his much-adored mother from lymphoma when she was still very young. She was a housewife and a mother and had

Occupations Linked with Immune System Cancers

Bartenders

Building caretakers

Cleaners

Cooks

Drivers

Electrical workers

Farmers

Hairdressers

Machinery fitters for metal processors

Painters

Pesticide applicators

Plumbers

Rubber workers

Tailors

Textile workers

Waiters

never previously worked with chemicals. So don't think that just because you don't work with chemicals you are not at risk. Considering the increase of chemical substances in our everyday lives, is it any wonder that these cancers are on the increase?

Chemicals and Substances That Trigger the Development of Immune System Cancers

Chemicals in household products (hair dyes, cosmetics)

Dusts

Energy sources (electricity, nuclear)

Environmental pollutants (PCBs, dioxin)

Medications (immunosuppressive drugs; treatments for rheumatoid arthritis, HIV)

Pesticides (organochlorines; organophosphates; carbamates; phenoxy acid herbicides or contaminants; dicamba; the herbicides 2,4-dichlorophenoxyacetic acid, mecoprop, and atrazine; the fungicide captan; the fumigant carbon tetrachloride)

Plastics (vinyl chloride, synthetic fabrics, phthalates)

Solvents (benzene)

Traffic-related air pollution (petroleum, petroleum products, engine exhausts)

Fighting Back Against Cancer

The good news is that there appears to be a great deal we can now all do to fight back. The ever-growing number of proven alternative and complementary methods by which we can successfully treat certain types of cancer opens up fresh hope for an increasing number of people who are receptive to a new way of thinking.

Further good news is that many of these new methods, such as lowering exposure to chemicals and detoxing, are in many cases able to slow down the development and spread of existing cancers. For instance, soluble fibers grab on to and remove some of the most potent and persistant chemical carcinogens from our bodies. These great detoxers can not only lower the risk of developing cancer (something that most conventional therapies don't even begin to tackle), they can actually suppress the growth and spread of tumors.

The three-step program in Part I is ideal for people wishing to avoid and actively lower their body's levels of cancer-exacerbating and -triggering chemicals. I think it's best to say that, like all cancer treatments, some work on certain cancers better than others. While it can be difficult to know whether you are one of the ones who will benefit from it, the act of avoiding cancer-causing chemicals and ensuring you are getting enough nutrients is a sensible precaution.

Supplements

The power of nutrients in preventing and suppressing cancer is such that now many doctors advocate cancer treatment methods based on nutritional techniques. Indeed, the use of nutrients in preventing, inhibiting, or delaying the progression of cancer is now somewhat confusingly referred to in mainstream medicine as *chemoprevention*.

Not only do nutrients, such as vitamins A, C, and E, and minerals zinc and selenium, directly kill cancer cells, but they also slow down the speed of cancerous growth, reducing the aggressiveness with and extent to which cancer cells invade the rest of the body. They can also prevent new cancers from forming. Other vitamins, vitamin D and the B group, possess powerful tumor-suppressive abilities. Minerals, such as magnesium, reduce the risk of death from cancer, and the essential oils with omega-3 fats, in addition to reducing the risk of cancer, inhibit cancer growth and reduce metastases.

These nutrients also offer protection from the wide range of cancer-causing chemicals we are regularly exposed to, as well as those used in chemotherapy. This can be seen in reduced treatment side effects and lower incidences of cancer and recurrences in those who have the highest levels of these nutrients in their diets and bodies.

The crazy thing is that when we get cancer, our need for nutrients to fight cancer is never greater, yet our intake of them tends to fall, due to reduced food intake, inadequate digestion, malabsorption, vomiting, and an increased nutrient demand as a consequence of cancer therapy. This has the unwanted effect of reducing the ability of cancer patients to fight back naturally, as their inbuilt cancer-fighting systems need a good supply of nutrients to work.

ALTERNATIVE AND COMPLEMENTARY TREATMENTS

There are now many specialist centers that successfully use the above methods to treat disease, such as the Environmental Health Center in Dallas, or the Unit for Integrative Medicine at the Sloane-Kettering Cancer Center in New York. These and other centers use a combination of the following methods to treat cancer: diet (more raw, uncooked foods), nutritional supplements, herbal and plant extracts with anticancer properties (like lycopene and soy products and fungi), counseling, relaxation techniques, exercise, and other methods. These places are also usually very happy to work with people who also want to use conventional forms of cancer therapy.

Their philosophy, like mine, is based around helping the body to rid itself of cancer. All treatments work on some cancers better than others, but the advantage of alternative treatments is that they are generally based on therapies designed to work with the body and therefore have much lower toxicities. Just because they don't make you feel ill, it doesn't mean that they are not fighting cancer cells.

CHAPTER 11

Multiple Chemical Sensitivity

MULTIPLE CHEMICAL SENSITIVITY (MCS), also known as environmental illness, is a condition where previous high exposure to a significant amount of solvents, pesticides, or other chemicals renders people hypersensitive to a wide range of unrelated, previously tolerated chemicals at very low levels that do not affect the general population at large.

This disease tends to affect women as well as people known to have increased contact with chemicals, such as industrial workers, populations exposed to certain combinations of chemicals (like the Gulf War veterans), communities with air or water contamination, and others with unique exposure to particular chemicals.

Symptoms range from headaches; poor concentration; lightheadedness; and depression to breathing difficulties; wheezing; asthma; sneezing; flu-like symptoms; ear, nose, and throat disturbances; gastrointestinal problems like diarrhea; musculoskeletal problems; and even heart and circulatory problems. Indeed, according to Professor William J. Rea, MD—author of the four-volume series of textbooks *Chemical Sensitivities,* who has treated more than 20,000 environmentally ill patients—chemicals can affect virtually every part of our bodies, they may manifest any symptom.

Normally, symptoms are triggered following exposure to one or more chemicals. Even seemingly innocuous and unrelated exposures, like a whiff of perfume or a puff of smoke, can bring about an almost immediate reaction, resulting in the rapid onset of a collection of widespread symptoms affecting many organ systems. There may also be continual background symptoms, such as fatigue or muscle cramps, partly due to a high existing level of body toxins.

This disease also appears to be very common, since a recent study carried out in the state of California by physicians specializing in environmental medicine revealed that not only 6 percent of the population sampled had MCS, but a whopping 15.9 percent of people reported being "allergic to or made sick by a number of everyday chemicals."

Unfortunately, we can only rely on estimates for the real number of people with this condition since few doctors even know about this disease, let alone are able to diagnose or treat it. An absence of training in medical school and a dearth of information on toxic chemicals and how to remove them from the body leaves most doctors totally blank about this condition. Only those trained in environmental medicine are able to recognize and treat it, which explains why approximately 40 percent of all those with MCS have had to consult ten or more medical practitioners before being diagnosed.

MCS

Multiple chemical sensitivity is thought to occur where someone's previous chemical exposure has taken them over a certain inbuilt safety threshold. Once this chemical capacity has been reached, any further chemical exposure results in symptoms. Not too surprisingly, symptoms can be so severe that they can successfully make the sufferer avoid any futher chemical contact.

There are many chemicals that can predispose a person to this condition. They include a mixture of the following: toxic metals (mercury, aluminum, lead), pesticides (all types including organophosphates and carbamates), organochlorines (DDT, PCBs, dioxin), solvents, plastics, and halogens (chlorine, fluorine and bromine, and their compounds).

Products That Can Trigger Chemical Reactions

Aerosol air freshener

Aerosol deodorant

Aftershave lotion

Cigar smoke

Cigarette smoke

Cleaning fluids

Colognes and perfumes

Diesel exhaust

Diesel fuel

Dry-cleaning fluid

Electrical devices

Floor cleaner

Furniture polish

Garage fumes

Gasoline exhaust

Hairspray

Insect repellent

Insecticide spray

Laundry detergent

Marking pens

(continued)

Products That Can Trigger Chemical Reactions

Nail polish and nail polish remover

Oil-based paint

Paint thinner

Perfumes in cosmetics and other products

Pesticides

Public restroom deodorizers

Shampoo

Tar fumes

Varnish and lacquer

GULF WAR SYNDROME

Many scientists now believe Gulf War Syndrome is a type of MCS. Unexplained symptoms reported by veterans of the first Gulf War with Iraq in 1991 have caused heated international debate. The symptoms reported include fatigue, skin rash, muscle and joint pain, headaches, loss of memory, shortness of breath, gastrointestinal and respiratory symptoms, and extreme sensitivity to commonly occurring chemicals. Interestingly, the key to the puzzle of Gulf War Syndrome (GWS) may be due to the particular combination of the numerous deadly chemicals that these soldiers were exposed to as a result of their posting.

It has been hypothesized by researchers at Duke University in North Carolina that the particular combination of pesticides, such as organophosphates and carbamates, along with the solvents and toxic metals and other chemicals in the anthrax and botulism vaccinations soldiers were injected with, could have brought about more nerve damage than any one of these substances could have done individually. This chemical cocktail could have acted as the initial trigger for developing MCS and could explain why veterans of the first Gulf War now have a significantly higher prevalence of symptoms suggestive of MCS than the equivalent non–Gulf War military personnel.

Treatments for MCS

Avoidance of all forms of chemicals, not only in foods and drinks but also in the environment, is one of the cornerstones to treatment. This includes avoiding not just the chemicals that trigger the sudden attacks but the entire range of chemicals, as they all put pressure on an already beleaguered and overloaded detoxification system.

As people with MCS tend to have higher levels of fat-soluble poisons (like organochlorine pesticides and solvents) than nonaffected people, detoxification is essential, as only by reducing the existing body burden of chemicals can the body improve its ability to deal with future ones.

The chemical avoidance and detox program as described in Part I is well suited for people with MCS. However, people with more severe symptoms should get individual treatment and be detoxed in a highly specialized unit, such as that found at the Environmental Center in Dallas, a place I would highly recommend. Their greater buildup of chemicals in combination with their damaged detoxification system means that they may need extra help in detoxing.

SUPPLEMENTS

Nutrient supplements play a critical role in treating this condition, as virtually everyone who has MCS is deficient in at least one essential nutrient. Sixty percent of people already taking supplements are known to be deficient in at least one essential nutrient. This high nutrient demand is mostly created by the increased nutritional needs created from a greater body burden of chemicals. Indeed, while the program in this book will be sufficient for most people, those with severe disease may need to get certain nutrients in much higher levels (usually vitamin C and other antioxidants) or even intravenously. This is best done under appropriate medical supervision.

Despite a need for sulfur in order to detox chemicals, many of those with MCS may have difficulty in dealing with MSM-sulfur or even possibly the sulfur-containing amino acids. So MSM-sulfur should be avoided, and when sulfur amino acids are taken, it should be done cautiously a week or two after the rest of the nutrient regime has been started, and stopped if they trigger a reaction. Lastly, the previously described detox reaction, which lasts for a day or two in most non-MCS sufferers, can go on for weeks in people with MCS before symptoms (such as tiredness and exacerbation of existing symptoms) start to improve, reflecting their reduced ability to process chemicals.

DIET

A diet of organic foods is preferable, as well as one that contains a good level of raw, unprocessed fruits and vegetables. These will help keep the body's pH level alkaline, something that helps to enhance chemical detoxification.

CHAPTER 12

Obesity and Musculoskeletal Disorders

WE ALL KNOW THAT THE FOOD we eat plays a major part in determining how we look and feel. However, few realize the effects that our ever-increasing exposure to toxic chemicals are having on making us heavier and damaging our body shape. I only discovered the full extent to which we are being affected myself several years ago when researching my first book, *The Body Restoration Plan.*

We all know that good looks and a great body are important in our highly image-conscious society. We also know that over the last few decades more and more people are not only gaining weight, with the number of overweight adults doubling over the last decade, but their bodies are actually changing shape. Few people have the hourglass figures so commonly seen in the old black-and-white movies.

Nowadays in addition to being overweight, women also tend to have thicker waists and thighs while men have more abdominal fat or paunch. While changes in the diet have partly contributed to these changes, few realize the extent of damage done to their weight and body shape by their continued exposure to ever-greater amounts of chemicals in their food and environment.

Our weight and shape is largely determined by our natural and highly evolved weight control systems. This is a complex network of systems made up of the brain, hormones, and metabolism that is designed to keep our weight stable throughout our lives. It acts as a natural "slimming system."

When researching my first book, which examines the effects chemicals have on our weight, I was absolutely staggered to learn the extent to which toxic chemicals appear to be able to damage virtually every part of our musculoskeletal system. It seems that our muscles, bones, and joints are prime targets for many dangerous toxins.

But what really made me sit up and take notice was the effect toxic chemicals had on the energy-producing mitochondria inside our tissues, which appear to take a major bashing from the most common chemical toxins. Understanding this gave me my first real insight into what was behind the hitherto little understood disease of chronic fatigue syndrome, also known as myalgic encephalomyelitis.

Whether you are a top athlete or have retired and want to maximize your mobility, this chapter is for you. The information here will help any and everyone interested in improving their fitness and energy levels and mobility. It will also tell you how cutting chemicals can also improve your health if you currently suffer from chronic fatigue syndrome, arthritis, or one of the many other rheumatic diseases linked to our exposure to chemicals.

How Chemicals Contribute to Weight Gain

What appears to be happening is that our natural slimming system is being poisoned by the toxic chemicals we encounter in our everyday lives, and this damage is making it increasingly difficult for our bodies to control their weight. The end result is that we gain weight in the form of fat and not muscle, as chemicals tend to cause muscles to shrink and body fat to accumulate.

The hormones that control our body shape are also targeted by the toxins. In men this damage equates to smaller muscles and more fat, particularly around the stomach. In women this appears to translate to more fat accumulating around the stomach, waist, and thighs.

Virtually all chemicals we are exposed to in our food and environment possess some sort of weight-altering effect, even at very low levels. These include a wide range of pesticides, medicines, toxic metals, plastics, solvents, environmental pollutants, and fire retardants. For example, pesticides: The deeper I looked into each of the dozens of different synthetic chemicals found as pesticide residues in food, the clearer it became to me that in addition to these chemicals being used for the purpose of killing a huge variety of different forms of life, some, such as the carbamates, were also being used to promote growth in animals and were even regularly used as medicines to treat a whole range of human illnesses, such as an overactive thyroid gland, and possessed a weight-gain side effect.

At low doses, organophosphates have also been used to fatten up animals by severely reducing their ability to use up existing fat stores. As the animals' fat-burning abilities slow down, they gain weight more quickly, since they can't burn off body fat as well as they previously could. Their food needs also fall, as less food appears to go further. Though the use of organophosphates as growth promoters has now been banned, these former weapons of mass destruction are still one of the most common pesticides, and therefore continue to be found as residues in many of our foods.

It really doesn't matter how you are exposed, whether it is from a can of fly spray or from pesticide residues in food. Once the chemicals get into your body, the chances are your weight-control systems will be damaged, making it just that little bit harder to lose weight in the future.

Another group of chemicals with very powerful weight-gain effects are the organochlorines. Studies show that the higher the level of these chemicals in the body, the greater the body weight will be. One animal study found one type of organochlorine, the pesticide and widespread environmental pollutant hexachlorobenzene (HCB), to possess such extreme fattening effects that when their food intake was cut by 50 percent animals treated with HCB still managed to gain more weight than did untreated animals on full rations! What's more, since the weight gained from organochlorines appears to be in the form of fat rather than muscle, body shape is also affected: making the body flabbier.

Plasticizers, like the phthalates, also possess this weight-gain effect, as do many other chemicals such as fire retardants and solvents, as can be seen in many published animal studies.

Musculoskeletal Health

You can't stop men from wanting more and stronger muscles and women from wanting to have firmer, more-toned muscles. This desire to enhance muscle size, strength, and tone is also shared by millions of athletes and sports competitors who compete to win. However, chemical exposure has the effect of causing muscles to shrink. This not only has implications for our body shape, but also for our overall health, especially as we age when poor muscle strength can cause you to become significantly less mobile.

Musculosketal health can be measured by three key factors: muscle size, muscle strength, and muscle endurance. Bigger muscles are a great indicator of someone's overall fitness. The maximum size to which our muscles can grow is largely predetermined by our genetic makeup and our hormones, so that even with all the exercise in the world, you can not build them up beyond a certain predestined size, not without the benefit of illegal and highly dangerous steroids.

While muscle strength depends to some extent on the amount of muscle you have, the strength of the contraction also depends on the maximum amount of energy your muscle can muster. Energy is created by tiny cylindrically shaped structures in cells called mitochondria, which are responsible for converting the food we eat into a molecular form of energy the whole body can easily use known as adenosine triphosphate (ATP). Due to our muscles' immense appetite for energy, they tend to be packed with millions of these energy-producing powerhouses. The number of mitochondria in our muscles and their efficiency ultimately determines how strong our muscles are. Our ability to keep these mitochondria supplied with food and to take away their waste products determines the degree of muscle endurance.

HOW CHEMICALS LOWER ENERGY
LEVELS AND DAMAGE MUSCLES

Unfortunately, the hormones that control the ultimate size of our muscles and our energy-producing mitochondria both appear to be exquisitely sensitive to and readily damaged by a wide range of chemical toxins, many of which are currently in our bodies. This ability to lower the natural production of hormones, such as testosterone, will reduce the size that our muscles can grow to, while the poisoning effect on mitochondria will not only reduce their overall numbers, but can dramatically impair their overall effectiveness in producing energy.

So our existing body burden of chemicals acts as a highly efficient drain on daily energy levels. Consequently, our bodies are actually producing far less energy than they were originally designed to. So while most of us get by on what we have, we are functioning way below our real capacity.

Worse still, chemical damage can also reduce the body's ability to produce the exact foods needed in order to fuel the mitochondria. So not only can chemicals reduce muscle size and strength, but they can

Chemicals That Damage Our Musculoskeletal System

Drugs (a large number of prescription medications, including over one dozen antibiotics, nonsteroidal anti-inflammatories, and anthelmintics)

Fluoride and fluoride products

Herbicides (for example 2,4-D)

Persistent environmental contaminants (PCBs, dioxin)

Pesticides (organophosphates, organochlorines, pentachlorophenol, along with many others)

Plastics

Solvents

Toxic metals

also lower muscle endurance by limiting production of the food supply or by speeding up the accumulation of cramp-inducing waste products such as lactic acid. In real life, this translates to smaller, weaker muscles that get exhausted more easily.

Lastly, chemicals also lower the levels of one of the brain's most important natural get-up-and-go hormones, dopamine. This dopamine-lowering action has the effect of reducing your energy drive so that you don't feel like going out to the gym or taking a walk, reducing your total amount of activity.

For example, the pesticides organophosphates and synthetic pyrethroids are commonly used in household bug-killing preparations as well as being found in our food as pesticide residues. Animals exposed to these chemicals suddenly become less active, not only moving less but also in performing fewer grooming and all other kinds of activities. The effect they have is of an invisible chemical cosh. It appears to be chemically induced nerve damage, produced by lowering the level of certain movement-activating hormones through the poisoning of energy-producing mitochondria, and in the case of organophosphates, from the muscle tissue actually dissolving. Many pesticides are deliberately designed to target mitochondria, as the stronger the ability of a chemical to poison the mitochondria, the more effective it is in killing.

Organochlorines are also big players in the energy-lowering chemical league. They actively reduce our tissues' ability to convert food into readily usable energy in the form of ATP. Not only does this affect energy production in our mitochondria, but it affects all the mechanisms used by our bodies to produce useful energy.

Toxic metals also produce this energy-inhibiting effect and damage mitochondria, lowering levels of ATP. Fortunately, mitochondria are very resilient, so a good detoxification and nutritional program can potentially restore your body to its full complement, enhancing muscle power and endurance. Gradually, as your levels of natural muscle-building hormones start to recover, they will stimulate new muscle growth. Detoxing will also help restore your production of muscle-growing hormones, allowing you to realize your full muscular potential. So if someone is on the brink of sporting success, detoxifying and reducing their body burden of these muscle-shrinking, energy-draining chemicals could give them a totally legal competitive edge; leaving their competitors with their muscles struggling under their toxic-chemical burden.

Detoxing and avoiding toxins as set out in Part I will also give the ordinary mortal bigger and stronger muscles and increased stamina. It will also help raise energy levels noticeably throughout the day.

Chronic Fatigue Syndrome or ME

Modern living takes its toll on most people's energy levels; however, for some, things have gone much further than just being tired all the time. They get so tired that they can hardly get out of bed, let alone go to work. Their lack of energy has gone well past the stage of being just a nuisance and now dominates all aspects of their lives. It can turn a previously active existence into a living nightmare. They have chronic fatigue syndrome (CFS), also known as ME (myalgic encephalomyelitis).

It is a complex illness characterized by incapacitating fatigue (experienced as exhaustion and extremely poor stamina), neurological problems, and a constellation of other diverse symptoms that can include poor sleeping patterns, recurrent sore throat, painful and aching muscles, painful joints, headaches, and post-exercise fatigue. These symptoms tend to wax and wane, but are very often severely debilitating and can last for several months or years on end.

Although no age group is excluded, CFS appears to target people between the ages of twenty and forty. Conservative estimates of the numbers of people affected by this extremely debilitating disease stand at 1.4 percent of certain populations.

CFS appears to be associated with a significant number of physical defects. Not only are energy-producing systems grossly impaired (such as fewer and more damaged energy-producing mitochondria being present in muscle tissue), there are markedly lower levels of energy production, greater buildup of waste products following exercise, and lower levels of energy-releasing and other important energy-controlling hormones. Together, these characteristics have given chronic fatigue syndrome its name.

While the fatigue element is clearly important, in the early days when this condition first established itself as a new entity, it was named myalgic encephalomyelitis because all the sufferers had some degree of brain damage. According to Dr. Byron Hyde, founder and chairman of the Nightingale Institute for Health and Environment, in Burlington, Vermont, which is dedicated to the study of myalgic encephalomyelitis/ chronic fatigue syndrome: "All ME patients have a scientifically measurable brain injury. Less than 5 percent of all patients examined have had a primary psychiatric or social cause for their illness"

Added to this is evidence for further abnormalities, such as widespread immune system damage. This diversity of damage readily accounts for the other numerous and seemingly disjointed symptoms commonly accompanying CFS. This injury appears to be caused by many factors, including infection (viral, fungal, and bacterial), various different mineral and vitamin deficiencies, and allergies or sensitivities to foods, pollutants, animal products, plant products, and chemicals.

CHEMICALS AND CHRONIC FATIGUE SYNDROME

Chemicals appear to play a very prominent role in the current CFS epidemic. To date, chemical exposure is the only factor known to bring about all the detectable disorders and symptoms associated with chronic fatigue syndrome. Chemicals are known to be potent damagers of every single part of the body involved in energy production and activity. This includes the brain and nerves (25 percent of all industrial chemicals are neurotoxins), hormones (energy releasing and muscle growing), muscles, mitochondria, and all aspects of tissue metabolism. Chemicals are also known immune-system poisons, increasing the risk of infection. No other single cause to date has been found to achieve this widespread degree of destruction.

The types of chemicals involved in CFS include all the usual ones, toxic metals (such as mercury), pesticides (which damage nerves, the brain, hormones, mitochondria, and the immune system), organochlorines (all types from DDT and PCBs to dioxin), solvents, halogens, certain prescribed drugs, and plastics.

The fact that CFS is a fairly recently identified disease whose emergence has coincided with our greater exposure to everyday toxic chemicals reinforces this connection. Indeed, the fact that many of these chemicals are now in our bodies at levels that appear to be producing all the signs and symptoms of CFS strengthens this association further.

For example, people with chronic fatigue syndrome also tend to have higher levels of organochlorines in their body tissues. Organochlorines are known to dramatically lower the ability of mitochondria to produce energy, in addition to their brain poisoning actions and their damage to energy releasing and controlling hormones, such as dopamine and catecholamines.

We also know that fatigue syndromes are particularly common in people who are occupationally exposed to pesticides, insecticides, and other chemicals. For example, chemically exposed veterans of the first Gulf War have much higher rates of CFS than nonexposed veterans. In addition, a recent study of sheep farmers revealed that the greater their exposure to organophosphates from the sheep dip, the greater their risk of developing all the symptoms of chronic fatigue syndrome.

Toxic metals, too, are known nerve, hormone, immune system, and mitochondrial poisons, among their many other toxic attributes. So it comes as no surprise that those with higher body levels of these substances, such as mercury (from fillings, vaccines, and contaminated seafoods), cadmium, and nickel, have a reduced ability to produce energy and are more likely to become fatigued and go on to develop CFS.

These chemical links get stronger as up to half of all the people with chronic fatigue have now been found to have a condition called chemical sensitivity (see chapter 11). Chemical sensitivity is a disorder where people appear to be abnormally sensitive to the presence of toxic chemicals at concentrations far lower than those which would normally cause a problem in the general population. This commonality is strongly reciprocated, as up to 40 percent of those with chemical sensitivities show all the symptoms of chronic fatigue syndrome. Indeed, it can often be very difficult to distinguish between these two disorders.

Fortunately, once these issues are addressed, there is a good chance that CFS can be successfully tackled. The program in Part I has been designed to help people with CFS/ME do what is necessary to detox and avoid chemicals so they can rebuild their life and regain their health.

Arthritis and Connective Tissue Diseases

The number of those with arthritis and other rheumatic conditions is rising, making this the leading form of disability today. Conventional wisdom states that all this is due to our aging population. To an extent this is true, as the greater the wear and tear the body is subjected to, the higher the risk of developing osteoarthritis. So it seems logical that the older one is, the more susceptible to this form of arthritis one will become. As the average age of our population increases, the overall incidence of osteoarthritis should follow suit.

However, not all forms of arthritis showing an upsurge in recent years are so strongly linked to an aging population, since the other important inflammatory musculoskeletal diseases have also been increasing. These include diseases known as rheumatoid arthritis (RA), psoriatic arthritis, inflammatory spondylitis, systemic lupus erythematosis (SLE), scleroderma, Sjogren's syndrome, and systemic sclerosis (SS), which tend to be found in a much younger sector of the population, striking victims between twenty and forty years of age.

Although, like osteoarthritis, they can affect our joints, the way in which they do it differs significantly. Rather than being the result of ordinary wear and tear, as in osteoarthritis, these conditions wreak their damage through inflammation caused by an abnormally overheated natural defense system, which is thought to be triggered by environmental damage (see chapter 5).

An understanding of why we develop these autoimmune disorders is vital if we are to have any chance of successfully dealing with them. Conventional medicine treats this problem, in effect, by trying to throw a bucket of cold water over the fight, to calm it down. It does this by us-ing highly toxic drugs that suppress the ability of our entire defense system to fight any invader, not just our own tissues. However, this method not only fails to tackle the cause of the problem, it also threat-ens our ability to deal with real invaders, such as harmful bacteria and other infections when they come along.

Initial observations first alerted scientists to the fact that those working with or exposed to a wide range of toxic chemicals tended to be more susceptible to developing autoimmune diseases. For instance, people who were exposed to the highest levels of mercury from having a mouthful of mercury-based dental fillings were more likely to develop one of the above autoimmune connective-tissue diseases than those with fewer or no fillings.

What seems to happen is that toxic chemicals increase the rate at which the body creates autoantibodies (see chapter 5). This ability of chemicals to start off this disastrous self-destruction process ap-pears to be aided and abetted by a combination of genetic vulnera-bility and poor nutritional status, as low body levels of vitamins and minerals, particularly magnesium, can also trigger production of auto-antibodies.

In revving up the immune system, these chemicals also increase the level of inflammation-creating substances, which ultimately increase the level of tissue inflammation. This is one of the factors triggering disease flare-ups and speeding up disease progression.

Even if your type of arthritis is not one of the autoimmune-type arth-ropathies and is caused by wear and tear (osteoarthritis), the presence of these pro-inflammatory chemicals in your body will work to worsen the inflammation in existing diseased joints while also increasing the chance of disease flare-ups.

To date, the list of chemicals that appear to trigger different forms of inflammatory arthritis and connective tissue disorders is very extensive and growing. They include substances from toxic metals used in dental fillings to solvents used in the dry-cleaning industry. There are dozens of "therapeutic" synthetic drugs that have also now been linked to auto-immune diseases.

Chemical Triggers of Connective Tissue Diseases

Antibiotics (penicillin, septrin, practolol)

Anticonvulsants (phenytoin, isoniazid, chlorpromazine, hydantoin, and primidone)

Antithyroid drugs (propylthiouracil, methylthiouracil, methyldopa, and cocaine)

Cancer drugs (bleomycin, pentazocine, and hydralazine)

Diesel exhaust particles

Environmental pollutants (PCBs, dioxin)

Estrogen

Fluorine

Hair dyes

Pesticides (DDT and organophosphates)

Solvents (vinyl chloride, epoxy resins, alcohol, benzene, trichloroethylene)

Steroids (procainamide and prednisone)

Toxic metals (mercury, cadmium, arsenic, lead, antimony, tin, cobalt, gold, silica, and silicone breast implants)

Xenoestrogens

How Chemicals Are Linked to Arthritis and Connective Tissue Diseases

Several famous artists, for example, Rubens, Renoir, and Dufy, are thought to have been early casualties of this particular form of chemical attack, possibly due to their love of bright and clear colors. They all suffered from rheumatoid arthritis, a disease known to be triggered by an exposure to toxic metals. Brighter and clearer color paints tended to be made up from toxic metals such as mercury, cadmium, arsenic, lead, antimony, tin, cobalt, manganese, and chromium, whereas the earth colors tended to contain less toxic ingredients, such as harmless iron and carbon compounds.

Analysis of the areas of various colors in randomly selected paintings by these artists compared to "control" artists (contemporary painters without rheumatic disease) suggests that Rubens and Renoir used significantly more bright and clear colors based on toxic metals and fewer earth colors. While their preference and increased use of these more vivid colors obviously helped them to enjoy extraordinary artistic success, it now seems that it could have come at a high price to their health. Artists today are not so exposed, but toxic metal contamination in food and drinking water exists.

In 1996, a citizens group in Nogales, Arizona, reported to the Arizona Department of Health their concerns about a possible excess of systemic lupus erythematosus (SLE) due to exposure to environmental contamination in the area. A study revealed that not only did they have a high incidence of people suffering from SLE, but that the people affected had been and were being exposed to raised levels of organochlorines and organophosphates in their polluted environment.

Another study in southwestern Ontario found an increased prevalence of systemic sclerosis in those who have more dental fillings. Yet another revealed that solvents are associated with various connective tissue diseases (systemic sclerosis, scleroderma, undifferentiated connective tissue disease, systemic lupus erythematosis, and rheumatoid arthritis), particularly systemic sclerosis.

Even the fluorine present in some forms of steroids given to people with rheumatoid arthritis is not only thought to trigger widespread bone demineralization, but also a worsening of the arthritis.

Restoring Your Weight and Musculoskeletal System

Detoxing opens up numerous safe and highly effective ways that you can readily increase your existing fitness, mobility, and energy levels whether you are an athlete or have had arthritis for years. Since these methods work by treating the causes of low energy, fatigue, muscle pain, and arthritis by removing toxic chemicals rather than by suppressing symptoms with potentially highly toxic drugs, they have to be a valid option. The detox program in Part I is well suited to help you regain your energy, mobility, and fitness.

SUPPLEMENTS

Supplements play a vital role in lowering the body burden of existing mobility-damaging, muscle-poisoning, and energy-grabbing toxins. Many also act as natural anti-inflammatories, which will help calm down existing disease flare-ups while preventing future episodes. They also work by giving the body the ability to kick out existing mobility-damaging toxins and reduce damage done by ones already present.

DIET

Fortunately, these toxin-induced body-shape-damaging effects can be reversed by following the three-step program described in Part I. If you want to know more about regulating your weight, look up my first book, *The Body Restoration Plan*. As well as explaining the problem in far greater detail, it will also provide you with extra support by explaining where the most fattening chemicals can be found in our environment and by giving you a selection of specially designed diet plans and recipes.

CHAPTER 13

Childhood Disorders

WHILE THE EFFECTS OF environmental toxins on adults are bad enough, the thought of the even-more-severe effects they are having on our children horrifies me. Although these next few pages only scratch the surface of this vast subject, my aim here is to introduce you to the immense health problems that chemicals are already bringing to the human race.

Among the 3,000 chemicals produced in highest volume (over 1 million pounds per year), only twelve have been adequately tested for their effects on the developing brain. This is a matter of great concern because the vulnerable fetuses and children are being exposed to untold numbers, quantities, and combinations of substances whose safety has never been established.

The problem stems from the fact that children are affected by much smaller levels of chemicals than those considered safe for adults. Even with chemicals that have been tested, the safety limits are based on adults' tolerances, which means that the unique needs of our children have been virtually ignored.

Children are not simply little adults. They lack a mature detoxification system that can process and expel the chemicals they are exposed to. Furthermore, because most of their body systems are still developing, the chemical poisoning of these systems brings about not only immediate damage but also increases the child's overall chances of developing a wide range of chemically related diseases in later life. To get an idea of the type of disease I am talking about, just go to the contents page.

In order for our future generations to survive and thrive, we all need to do our part as parents to protect our children from the accompanying hazards. While the number of childhood disorders linked to exposure to toxic chemicals is extensive, I have decided to concentrate on the following increasingly common behavioral and learning problems, which tend to start in childhood, namely: attention deficit disorder (ADD) or attention-deficit/hyperactivity disorder (ADHD), autism, and learning difficulties.

ADHD and ADD

ADHD is thought to affect approximately 2 to 3 million children in the United States. Some children appear to have a greater problem with hyperactivity-type symptoms, others with poor concentration, and the rest have a combination of both. Although these symptoms tend to lessen during adolescence, a minority carry on to be afflicted by the same symptoms into mid-adulthood, where in many cases ADHD is also associated with anxiety, mood, and other disruptive disorders, as well as substance abuse. Poor concentration on its own is referred to as ADD or attention deficit disorder.

At the heart of these symptoms appears to be a marked inability of the brain to produce enough of the neurotransmitters/hormones known as catecholamines (see chapter 6). These vital energizing substances, which are created from dopamine (see Parkinson's disease), are critical in energizing the body, initiating movement, and improving concentration, among other things (see weight control). Low levels of brain catecholamines result in hyperactivity and inattention. Ritalin, which increases the release of catecholamines, appears to calm previously disruptive children down, but has a raft of accompanying toxic side effects.

Recent imaging studies have revealed that certain parts of the brains of ADHD children tend to be abnormally smaller than those of normal children, while other parts appear to be larger. Those affected by ADHD also appear to have a lower blood flow to the brain. This is of great concern as something out there appears to be powerful enough not only to change the way the brain works but also to change its very structure in millions of children. So what could be doing this? You guessed it—toxic chemicals.

CHEMICALS AND ADHD

While genetics appear to play some role in triggering ADHD, the sheer increase in the number of those developing this condition would suggest that the factors responsible reflect recent changes to our diet and environment. Since an estimated 25 percent of the industrial chemicals in our environment are known neurotoxins—that is, they are known to poison nerve and brain cells—these would seem to be an obvious source of the problem.

If you delve a little deeper you will see that not only are chemicals known to possess a powerful ability to change the shape of developing brains, but the vast majority of synthetic chemicals appear to damage and lower the level of catecholamines (the hormones epinephrine and norepinephrine) and dopamine produced by brain cells. Indeed, some toxic chemicals are so good at creating ADHD-like symptoms, they are even used to produce animal models of the disease for research purposes, such as an artificial chemical used to block brain dopamine production (6-hydroxydopamine). It is therefore easy to understand how the ever-increasing exposure of our children to these known neurodevelopmental chemical toxins could be playing a major role in the ADHD epidemic.

Unfortunately, some of the chemicals most strongly linked to ADHD are those commonly found in the body of every prospective parent. Consequently, babies are exposed to these toxins before they are even conceived. For instance, the toxic metals, lead and mercury, and the environmental pollutants, PCBs and DDT—all chemicals associated with ADHD—are already found in many people at levels known to damage brain development in unborn babies.

It is known that the developing brain is exquisitely sensitive to mercury. One study showed that the greater the amount of mercury in contaminated foods eaten by a pregnant woman, the greater the attention, language, and memory problems her child had by the age of seven. Lead levels also appear to be strongly linked to ADHD as the higher the level of lead in a child's blood or hair, the more likely the child is to get ADHD symptoms. Yet toxic metals continue to be given to children in vaccines at levels hundreds of times over the "safe" daily exposure levels. While mercury has been removed from regular childhood vaccinations, it is still used in other vaccines children might be given. Aluminum is still present in many regular childhood vaccines.

Since the universally found organochlorine contaminants known as PCBs can powerfully and permanently lower the amount of catecholamines produced in the brain, it is no surprise that the number of children developing ADHD is on the increase. Indeed, mothers who have higher body levels of other catecholamine-depleting toxins, such as the commonly found organochloride pesticide known as DDT and its metabolite DDE, are also more likely to have children affected by ADHD.

Childhood exposure to other chemicals, such as pesticides commonly found in the diet, is also known to cause behavioral problems such as inattention, low IQ, and poor memory. Many pesticides have powerful dopamine- and catecholamine-hormone lowering effects, and indeed are actually used for this purpose.

Perhaps the best known connection between hyperactivity and chemicals is from food additives, colorings, and flavorings. Many studies have now demonstrated that children with ADHD show dramatic improvements after food colorings, additives, and flavorings in their diet are lowered.

So although ADHD is known to be a complex disorder, triggered by a number of different factors, it seems that lowering future exposure to chemicals in combination with removing existing ones from the body by way of a good detox program in which supplements play an important role, is an effective drug-free way of starting to tackle symptoms naturally.

Autism

Few childhood disorders are more emotionally distressing than autism. The combination of socially aloof behavior, a reduced ability to communicate, and an inability to integrate with other family members can push even the strongest child-parent bond to its limits. The effects on the family can be devastating, with siblings getting less attention and the parents' own relationship suffering, resulting in a higher divorce rate. So every case of this distressing disorder is a tragedy not only for the child but also for the whole family.

Until very recently, autism has been exceedingly uncommon and the previous medical view has been that it was caused by a genetic disorder. However, over the past few decades, the number of children developing autism has shot through the roof. For instance, in America, for every one case of autism in 1993, there are now eight. This is powerful evidence that the situation has dramatically worsened.

Young children with autism tend to have impaired language development. They have difficulty expressing needs (often using gestures instead of words) and may laugh, cry, or show distress for unknown reasons. Some may develop abnormal patterns of speech that lack intonation and expression and may obsessively repeat words or phrases. In general, autistic children do not express interest in other people and often prefer to be alone. They may resist changes in their routine, repeat actions (e.g., turn in circles, flap their arms) over and over, and engage in self-injurious behavior (e.g., biting or scratching themselves, or banging their head). These changes in behavior are associated with many of the following factors:

➤ Most have indications of brain dysfunction.
➤ Approximately half have abnormal electroencephalograms (EEGs).

➤ More than 25 percent of autistic children and adolescents have abnormally low levels of the neurotransmitter serotonin in the brain.

➤ Abnormalities in body levels of catecholamines are commonly found.

➤ The immune system appears to be damaged in many of those affected, with autoimmune disorders a particular problem (antibodies against myelin proteins are frequently found).

➤ Malabsorption problems such as a leaky gut and dysbiosis are rife.

➤ Impaired detoxification of chemicals was found in 100 percent of the autistic patients tested in one study. Damage to sulphur metabolism commonly associated with detoxification disorders is also linked to gut malabsorption problems.

➤ Food intolerances are frequently present (particularly dairy and gluten-containing foods).

CHEMICALS AND AUTISM

The prevailing view is that autism is caused by a genetic predisposition together with a series of early environmental shocks to the developing nervous system, mainly from toxic chemicals such as those found in contaminated foods, polluted water, and polluted air. The children who develop autism tend to be those who are exposed to higher levels of these chemicals (particularly toxic metals such as aluminum, mercury, pesticides, and certain medicinal drugs like thalidomide and antiepilepsy medications) at certain stages of their development, but are less able to break them down.

This reduced detoxing ability could be due to being exposed at a very young age, when the immune system is relatively immature; from a reduced genetic ability to deal with chemicals; or insufficient levels of detoxing nutrients. It could also help explain why autistic children tend to have a higher body burden of toxic chemicals, in particular toxic metals. Autism could then arise following a final trigger such as an infection, a vaccination, or something else.

This powerful chemical link is reflected in the fact that chemicals have been used to create animal models of autism. Laboratory rats are exposed to valproic acid—a medicinal drug for treating epilepsy or thalidomide. The rats then go on to develop many of the brain abnormalities associated with autism in humans.

There is also a strong connection between all forms of vaccinations and autism. A U.S. study found that children who received vaccines containing a preservative called thimerosal, which is almost 50 percent mercury, were more than twice as likely to develop autism than children who did not. Although mercury has been removed from regular childhood vaccines due to growing safety worries, it is still present in other vaccines children might get. Aluminum, another toxic metal, is still present in childhood and many other vaccines, in addition to a whole raft of other toxic chemicals and live viruses.

When working at the Royal Free Hospital in London, Dr. Andrew Wakefield first made the connection between vaccination and autism after he saw an increasing number of children with a previously unknown bowel disorder (now known as ileocolonic lymphonodular hyperplasia) in a group of children with autism. Of forty-eight children who had developed autism just after being given the MMR vaccine (which, incidently, does not contain mercury), forty-six exhibited these same bowel abnormalities. In his view, the sheer number of children showing up with this previously extremely uncommon bowel disorder, along with autistic tendencies that started soon after vaccination, was more than just coincidence.

Together with his colleague Dr. Andrew Shattock, Wakefield postulated that an attenuated strain of the measles virus caused a reaction in the bowel wall that damaged it and made it more porous. Wakefield then speculated that the associated deficiencies in vitamin B_{12} from a reduced ability to absorb this nutrient from food contributed to the autistic regression seen in those children, since this nutrient is essential for the normal development of the central nervous system.

Autism-linked bowel problems can also be triggered by a high exposure to chemicals and a reduced ability to deal with them as the bowel becomes more damaged and leaky (see chapter 7). This causes inadequately digested foods (in the form of peptides) to escape into the bloodstream, then eventually enter the brain, upsetting normal functioning. Foods known to trigger this effect include those containing gluten (wheat, rye, barley, and oats), and milk and dairy products.

In conclusion, it seems that a number of chemical factors play a role in triggering the onset of autism. In the case of MMR-triggered autism, the virus in this vaccine could be the final straw, triggering autism in a child who has already been damaged by previous exposure to chemicals from vaccines and the environment. Major improvements can be made. They center around a detox program, a good rounded supplement program, and a diet low in gluten and dairy foods.

Dyslexia

It is now estimated that 10 percent of the population of the United States and United Kingdom suffer to some extent with dyslexia and that 4 percent are severely affected. Dyslexia, a reduced ability or inability to read or spell, is found in families across the full range of socioeconomic backgrounds. In practice, the term *dyslexia* tends to be used as an umbrella term for a number of related disorders of common origins, such as:

➤ Dyspraxia (problems with learning and with planning and executing sequences of coordinated movements; for example, eating with a spoon, riding a bike, or speaking clearly)
➤ Dyscalculia (problems with numbers)
➤ Dysgraphia (problems with handwriting)

Dyslexia literally means the inability to master the written word. It is usually described as having "word blindness." A dyslexic brain has problems in seeing, understanding, or recognizing some words. The result is that some dyslexics are unable to read well, to write fluently, or to spell competently, despite strenuous efforts made on the part of both teacher and learner.

Dyslexia symptoms are also found in similar disorders such as attention-deficit/hyperactivity disorder (ADHD). Interestingly, this could be more than just coincidence, as these conditions share many other features, such as abnormal levels of brain neurotransmitters such as catecholamines, abnormal energy metabolism in the brain, abnormal-sized structures in the brain, increased brain symmetry in areas where it should be more asymmetrical, and also the reverse. So what is thought to cause this problem?

CHEMICALS AND DYSLEXIA

Although there is a powerful genetic predisposition to dyslexia, the increase in numbers of those with dyslexia symptoms is probably due to the huge amount of toxic chemicals in the environment, which are known to damage our developing nervous systems. This form of damage results in abnormal wiring between different parts of the brain, underdevelopment or overdevelopment in other parts of the brain, and an imbalance in the brain's ability to create neurotransmitters. The upshot of this is that the damaged brain cannot process information as it was designed to do, resulting in the above-mentioned reading and learning problems.

While it is difficult to point fingers at any particular chemical, many are known to be more strongly linked to dyslexia than others. For instance, toxic metals are well known to destroy nerves. There is a close correlation between the level of mercury that children are exposed to in the womb and the degree of language and memory deficits that result. In other words, the higher the level of mercury, the greater the degree of dyslexia. Other metals, such as cadmium, lead, and aluminum, also tend to be found in much higher levels in dyslexic children.

Other environmental contaminants, such as PCBs (found in high levels in fish and animal products), are known to produce features common to dyslexia, such as abnormal levels of brain catecholamines and an altered brain shape and symmetry. Organochlorine pesticides, such as DDT and a wide number of other pesticides and solvents, can also damage the energy metabolism in certain parts of the brain involved in reading. Increased damage to the energy production in these

areas could explain why reading causes these parts of the brain to become more fatigued in dyslexics, compared to nondyslexics.

Looking on the positive side, it is very possible to considerably improve the situation in a developing child by lowering their future exposure to nerve-killing chemicals while simultaneously lowering the existing
levels of chemicals in their bodies, as this will help prevent future damage. While some of this damage is permanent, such as a reduction in
IQ if the child affected is under the age of six (i.e. while the brain is
most rapidly developing), it is never too late to reduce a child's chemical burden in order to restore some of the damage done. Recent studies now reveal that the brain keeps developing well into the late forties.

In addition to a good detox plan that includes a good level of toxin-
binding soluble fiber and essential nutrients, chelation therapy has been
used to significantly benefit the 1 to 2 percent of preschool children
whose blood lead levels are 250 micrograms per liter or higher. Chelation
therapy is a treatment that uses substances such as 2, 3-demercapto-
succinic acid (DMSA), dimercaptopropanesulfonate (DMPS), and eth-
ylenediaminetetraacetic acid (ETDA) to bind toxic metals. This needs
to be done under medical supervision due to the potential side effects.
While chelation therapy is potentially useful in many children with
very high levels of toxic metals in their system, a good detox program
using nutrients and soluble fiber will work just as effectively and be
safer. Such a program will need to be followed for a few months as it
takes time for the metals to be removed from the system.

Tackling Childhood Health

By taking care to reduce harmful toxins, you have the unique ability
to give your children the best start in life that a parent can give their
child, good health. Whether your child is a toddler or teenager, it's
never too late to improve their health.

Ideally, to protect our children we need to start lowering their exposure
to chemicals at the earliest possible stage. This means that prospective
parents should embark on a detox program even before they try to con-

ceive. Then during pregnancy the mother should reduce her exposure to all forms of chemicals, particularly during the first three months. Once their child is born, parents need to ensure that sensible efforts are made to reduce all forms of chemical exposure. These efforts include avoiding concentrated forms of chemicals such as pesticide sprays, peeling fruit and vegetables, eating more organic foods, filtering water, etc. In other words, the same precautions that I have recommended for adults.

SUPPLEMENTS

Nutrients play an important role in preventing chemically related damage and optimizing our health. However, the combination of less nutritious, increasingly processed food, together with a less varied diet means that the vast majority of children, from babyhood upward, are now not getting the nutrients they need to grow and develop properly, let alone to defend their bodies against the onslaught of toxic chemicals. Not only do chemicals increase our children's need for certain nutrients in order to process them, but many chemicals themselves increase nutrient deficiencies by reducing nutrient absorption. For instance, lead exposure promotes iron deficiency. If you combine this with the fact that children with iron deficiencies are much more vulnerable to lead poisoning, it makes sense to ensure that children at risk from lead poisoning are given a sufficient level of iron. Other nutrients which prevent lead poisoning by reducing its absorption or by accelerating its safe removal from the body are magnesium (vitally important), calcium, vitamin C, zinc and MSM-sulphur.

As you can see, the good news is that this situation can be easily remedied by making sure you give your children the nutrients they need in the form of supplementation. Indeed, since mothers who take nutrients during pregnancy lower their child's risk of developing childhood cancer as well as a large number of other diseases, it is never too early to start.

The program has been written for adults, however it can be adapted for children. Using supplements designed for children, follow dosing guidelines on the side of the supplement packet to get the appropriate level of nutrients for your child.

DIET

We are what we eat. This is particularly true for children. With time at a premium, it can be only too easy to give children the food they so crave, the highly processed, sugar- and fat-filled variety. As a parent it is up to you to ensure that they get as much fresh and uncooked fruits and vegetables as possible.

This is particularly important for children with diseases like autism. Their bowel complaints make it not only more difficult for them to absorb nutrients from food, but it also causes certain foods to aggravate their behavioral symptoms. These foods, such as those containing gluten, and milk and dairy products, should be severely restricted, which could result in significant behavioral benefits. If this is done, it is essential to ensure the body is getting enough nutrients, as cutting out a major food group can cause imbalances in the overall nutrient intake.

Children at risk from lead poisoning from a contaminated environment should eat a low-fat diet in combination with a good amount of protein, as this will lower the amount of lead absorbed. Lastly, frequent hand washing, especially before meals, significantly helps to lower the amount of lead dust a child will ingest.

Resources

Visit Dr. Paula Baillie-Hamilton's Web site at www.slimmingsystems.com

Environmental Medicine

The American Academy of Environmental Medicine
7701 East Kellogg
Suite 625
Wichita, KS 67207
(316) 684 5500
www.aaem.com
This organization will give you the names of specialists in your area.

The Environmental Health Center
8345 Walnut Hill Lane
Suite 220
Dallas, TX 75231
(214) 368 4132
www.ehcd.com
An excellent hospital that treats people with environmentally triggered illnesses.

Mercury-Free Dentistry

The International Academy of Oral Medicine and Toxicology
8297 Champions Gate Boulevard
Suite 193
Champions Gate, FL 33896
(863) 420-6373
Email: info@iaomt.org
www.iaomt.org
If you go to this Web site, the excellent but chilling "Smoking Teeth" presentation by Dr. Kennedy makes essential viewing.

Detoxing Supplements and Foods

Shaklee Corporation
www.shaklee.com
This multilevel marketing company sells great nutrients, herbals, and a wide range of household products to help you detox.

Whole Foods Market
www.wholefoods.com
"The world's largest natural and organic foods supermarket," it also sells supplements.

New Chapter
(800) 543-7279
Email: info@new-chapter.com
"Delivering the wisdom of nature." Vitamins, minerals, herbs, probiotics, MycoMedicinal mushroom products. A small company dealing in high-quality, organically sourced products.

Organic Living

The range of organic products on the market is increasing at a tremendous pace. There are many books available that contain this information on finding a range of organic products in an ever-expanding number of countries. In addition, the Internet is a very good source of information.

Natural Home Products
www.naturalhomeproducts.com
A company that sells organic carpets, flooring, bedding, children's necessities, and other household goods.

Natural Shop
www.shopnatural.com
A source of natural and organic products.

Grass Roots Natural Goods
www.grassrootsnaturalgoods.com
A company specializing in natural hemp clothing, bags, jewelry, footwear, organic cotton apparel, household and body-care products.

Chemical Information Web Sites

Shirley's Wellness Café
www.shirleys-wellness-cafe.com
An excellent health resource for humans and pets. Shirley's Wellness Café is well worth a visit.

Silent Spring Institute
www.silentspring.org
Silent Spring Institute is a nonprofit scientific research organization dedicated to identifying the links between the environment and women's health, especially breast cancer.

Fluoride Action Network
www.fluorideaction.org
Fluoride Action Network is an international coalition working to end water fluoridation and alert the public to fluoride's health and environ-

mental risks. Contains reams of information about ways in which fluoride can damage health.

Dr. Mercola
www.mercola.com
Dr. Mercola has a very interesting Web site which contains an excellent section on mercury toxicity in the "dental corner."

Recommended Reading

Beaumont, P. *Pesticides, Policies and People: A Guide to the Issues.* London: The Pesticides Trust, 1993.

Caton, Helen, Harold Buttram, and Damien Downing. *The Fertility Plan: A Holistic Program for Conceiving a Healthy Baby.* New York: Fireside Books, 2000.

Clarke, A., et al. *Living Organic: Easy Steps to an Organic Family Lifestyle.* London: Time-Life Books, 2001.

Dadd, Debra Lynn. *Home Safe Home: Protecting Yourself and Your Family from Everyday Toxics and Harmful Household Products.* New York: Jeremy P. Tarcher/Putnam, 1997.

Erasmus, U. *Fats that Heal, Fats that Kill.* Vancouver: Alive Books, 1987/1994.

Heaton, S. *Organic Farming, Food Quality and Human Health.* Bristol, England: Soil Association, 2001.

Holford, P. *The Optimum Nutrition Bible,* London: Piatkus, 1998.

McTaggert, Lynne, ed. *The Medical Desk Reference.* London: What Doctors Don't Tell You Publications Ltd., 2000.

Rea, W. *Chemical Sensitivity, Vols 1–4.* Boca Raton: CRC Press, 1992–96.

Teitelbaum, Jacob. *From Fatigued to Fantastic!: A Proven Program to Regain Vibrant Health.* New York: Avery, 2001.

Glossary

adrenaline (epinephrine) One of the most important slimming and energy-giving hormones we possess. It is easily damaged by toxic chemicals.

aduvants Aduvants are materials, such as heavy metals, that are added to one or more chemicals to enhance activity or performance.

allergy An abnormally heightened reaction an individual displays to a foreign substance or a substance perceived as foreign.

amino acids The basic building blocks from which proteins are made.

antioxidants Substances that are able to effectively neutralize and soak up harmful free radicals. Examples include vitamin A and beta-carotene, vitamins C and E, zinc, selenium, coenzyme Q10, and the amino acid glutathione.

asthma A breathing disorder associated with airway obstruction, marked by recurrent attacks of shortness of breath, with wheezing due to spasmodic contraction of the main airways.

attention deficit/hyperactivity disorder (ADHD) A behavior disorder originating in childhood, the essential features of which are signs of developmentally inappropriate inattention, impulsivity, and hyperactivity.

autism A disorder beginning in childhood marked by the presence of markedly abnormal or impaired development in social interaction and communication and a markedly restricted repertoire of activity and interest.

autoimmune diseases Diseases that are characterized by the production of antibodies that react against the body's own tissues.

carbamates A class of very widely used pesticides, added to food because of their ability to kill funguses.

chelation The solubilization and removal from the body of accumulated toxic metals, especially from nerve and brain tissue, using nutrients such as MSM-sulfur, magnesium, vitamin C, calcium, iron, and soluble fiber. A chelation detox, which requires medical supervision, uses synthetic substances that are not currently approved by the FDA to bind to toxic metals.

chronic fatigue syndrome A syndrome characterized by persistent or recurrent fatigue, diffuse musculoskeletal pain, sleep disturbances of six months' duration or longer.

colitis Inflammation of the colon.

connective tissue disorder A group of disorders characterized by abnormalities in one or more of the types of connective tissue, for example, collagen, elastin, or the mucopolysaccharides that effectively hold or glue the body together.

detoxification The removal of toxic substances from the body by the body's waste disposal systems.

diabetes Inability to control blood sugar levels.

dysbiosis An imbalance between the good and harmful bacteria in the digestive system that could predispose to disease.

dyslexia An impaired ability to understand written and printed words or phrases despite intact vision.

eczema An itchy, lumpy skin condition characterized by thickening of the skin, redness, small vesicles (fluid-filled spots), crusting, and weeping.

estrogens Female hormones that promote female physical characteristics.

free radicals These particles are produced in cells in the normal process of energy creation and damage and age all the tissues they are created in. Pesticides, smoking, exhaust fumes, pollution, infections, burned foods, fried foods, and sunburn all increase free radical production.

fungicide A chemical that destroys fungus.

glutathione An amino acid that is essential in breaking down toxic chemicals.

hayfever A seasonal type of allergy to pollen and other substances, otherwise known as allergic rhinitis, marked by red, itchy, and watery eyes.

halogens A group of similar elements in the periodic table including fluorine, chlorine, bromine, and iodine.

herbicide A chemical that is toxic to plants and is commonly used as a weed killer.

hormones Natural substances that act as internal messengers in our bodies. They are released from one part of our bodies and then carried around in the body fluids to another part, which they then stimulate.

hypertension Persistently high blood pressure. Currently accepted threshold levels are 140 for systolic and 90 for diastolic pressure.

inflammatory bowel disease Diseases that cause irritation and ulcers in the intestinal tract. Crohn's disease and ulcerative colitis are the most common inflammatory bowel diseases.

insecticide A substance used to kill insects.

insulin A hormone, the main role of which is to control blood sugar levels.

irritable bowel syndrome This condition includes a group of gastro-intestinal symptoms for which a cause is officially not known. It is characterized by a combination of abdominal pain and altered bowel function.

magnesium An essential mineral for protecting the body against toxic heavy metals. Usually deficient in people's diets, and low levels are associated with low energy, high blood pressure, and childhood learning and behavioral problems. Particularly good at ridding the body of lead.

mineral An inorganic substance that occurs naturally and is needed by the human body in small quantities for good health.

mitochondrion The part of a cell that transforms foods into a usable source of energy. Mitochondria are readily damaged by toxic chemicals.

multiple chemical sensitivity A disorder characterized by immediate recurrent symptoms in one or more of the major organ systems in response to demonstrable exposure to many chemical compounds at doses below those established in the general population to cause harmful effects.

multiple sclerosis A nerve disorder mainly affecting young adults and characterized by destruction of myelin (fatty sheath surrounding nerve fibers) in the brain.

neurotransmitter A chemical messenger (e.g., dopamine or serotonin) used to transmit or prevent messages being relayed through nerves or between nerves in the central nervous system and other types of cells.

nutrient A substance that provides nourishment essential for the maintenance of life and growth.

omega-3 oils The omega-3s are one of two families of fatty acids that are essential for growth and development and cannot be made by the body. Most people tend to be deficient in this nutrient and require supplementation. Our bodies function best when there is a balance of omega-3s and 6s in our diet.

omega-6 oils The omega-6s are one of two families of essential fatty acids needed for growth and development that cannot be made by the body. Most people tend to get enough of this nutrient in their diets.

organic In 2000, Secretary of Agriculture Dan Glickman announced the national standards for the production, handling, and processing of organically grown agricultural products. Essentially, the organic standard offers a national definition for the term "organic," and details the methods, practices, and substances that can be used in producing and handling organic crops and livestock, as well as processed products. The guidelines establish clear organic labeling criteria, and specifically prohibit the use of genetic engineering methods, ionizing radiation, and sewage sludge for fertilization.

organic chemicals Substances derived from living organisms, containing carbon.

organic solvents A solvent is a liquid that dissolves a solute. The solvent is the component of the solution that is present in greater amount. Organic solvents include substances such as benzene, tetrachloroethylene, and turpentine. They are usually flammable materials and may pose certain physical and chemical hazards.

organochlorines A number of organic chemicals that contain the substance known as chlorine. These types of compounds are not found to occur naturally. Due to our inability to remove them from our bodies, and their longevity, they tend to be extremely persistent in the body as well as being toxic. This varied group includes chemicals known as DDT, PCBs, dioxin, and lindane.

organohalogens A number of artificial and highly toxic compounds, which include the organochlorines, pesticides, PCBs, and the PBB fire retardants. They are particularly persistent and toxic and are not found in nature. Their difficult molecular shape (because of the halogenated component), often makes it impossible for our bodies' waste disposal systems to see and remove them.

organophosphates Synthetic organic compounds containing phosphorus, which include highly toxic pesticides and nerve gases.

Parkinson's disease A progressive, degenerative brain disease characterized by a tremor that is most marked at rest, a tendency to fall backward, stiff and rigid limbs, stooped posture, slowness of voluntary movements, and a mask-like facial expression.

PBBs (polybrominated biphenyls) Organohalogen compounds that contain bromine. These substances are not found in nature and include a number of highly stable heat-resistant compounds—and because of these qualities they are commonly used as fire retardants. However, due to our relative inability to remove them from our bodies, our bodily levels of these chemicals tend to accumulate throughout our lives.

PCBs (polychlorinated biphenyls) Although the manufacture of these types of organochlorines is now banned, these very stable and persistant organochlorines are still found in our environment and our bodies.

pentachlorophenol A highly toxic chemical formerly commonly used as a herbicide and fungicide. Due to marked toxicities, its use is now restricted.

pesticide A substance used for destroying insects or other organisms harmful to cultivated plants or to animals and humans.

phthalates A group of chemical compounds added to plastics to increase their flexibility. They have been banned for use in toys and cosmetics in some European countries due to their toxicity.

plasticizers Chemicals added to plastics (synthetic resins) to produce or promote flexibility and to reduce brittleness, such as phthalates.

pollutants Substances that pollute or contaminate the environment, especially harmful chemical or waste material discharged into the atmosphere and water, including gases, particulate matter, pesticides, radioactive isotopes, sewage, organic chemicals and phosphates, solid wastes, and many others.

scleroderma A chronic disorder marked by hardening and thickening of the skin. It may be localized or may affect the whole body.

Sjogren's syndrome A chronic inflammatory autoimmune disorder that is characterized by dry eyes, dry mouth, and arthritis.

stroke A sudden loss of brain function due to a blood clot or a bleed in or from a blood vessel in the brain.

supplement A substance taken to remedy the deficiencies in a person's diet.

synthetic chemical A substance made by chemical synthesis, especially to imitate a natural product. These synthetic chemicals or substances do not exist in nature.

systemic lupus erythematosus An autoimmune disorder characterized by periodic episodes of inflammation of joints, tendons, organs, and other connective tissues.

testosterone A hormone that controls the development of male sexual characteristics. It is very vulnerable to chemical damage.

thyroid hormones A group of hormones that regulate growth and development by altering the body's metabolic rate.

trans fat An unhealthy fat found in fried foods, cookies, crackers, and donuts, that are created by the hydrogenation of healthy fats such as corn or soybean oil.

vitamin Any of a group of compounds essential for normal growth and nutrition and required in small quantities in a person's diet because they cannot be created by the body.

VOCs (volatile organic chemicals) Organic compounds that evaporate readily at normal pressures and temperatures. Organic chemicals are widely used as ingredients in household products. Paints, varnishes, and wax all contain organic solvents, as do many cleaning, disinfecting, cosmetics, wood preservatives, air fresheners, dry-cleaned clothes, aerosol sprays, fuels, degreasing, and hobby products. All these products can release organic compounds when you are using them and to some degree when stored.

xenobiotics Foreign or unnatural compounds or chemicals (i.e., those that do not exist in nature).

xenoestrogen An unnatural artificial chemical that mimics the actions of natural estrogens (female hormones).

References

CHAPTER 1. The Perils of a Polluted World

Baillie-Hamilton, P. Chemical Toxins: A Hypothesis to Explain the Global Obesity Epidemic. *Journal of Alternative and Complementary Medicine* 2002; 8(2): 185–92.

CHAPTER 3. Step 2. Seven-Day Desludge Diet

Vidal, J. Scientists Suspect Health Threat from GM Maize. *The Guardian* (London). 27 February 2004.

CHAPTER 5. Immune System Diseases

Alexander, J. W. Immunoenhancement via Enteral Nutrition. *Annals of Allergy, Asthma & Immunology* 1993; 128(11): 1242–45.

Dewailly, E. et al. Susceptibility to Infections and Immune Status in Inuit Infants Exposed to Organochlorines. *Environ Health Perspective* 2000; 108(3): 205–11.

Drouet, M. et al. [Mercury—Is It a Respiratory Tract Allergen?] *Allergie et Immunologie* 1990; 22(3): 84–88.

Hoppin, J. A. et al. Chemical Predictors of Wheeze among Farmer Pesticide Applicators in the Agricultural Health Study. *American Journal of Respiratory and Critical Care Medicine* 2002; 165(5): 683–89.

King, L. E. Zinc Deficiency in Mice Alters Myelopoiesis and Hematopoiesis. *Journal of Nutrition* 2002; 132(11): 3301–307.

McKeever, T. M. et al. The Importance of Prenatal Exposures on the Development of Allergic Disease: A Birth Cohort Study Using the West Midlands General Practice Database. World Health Organization (WHO) 2002; 166(6): 827–32.

Peden, D. Pollutants and Asthma: Role of Air Toxics. *Environmental Health Perspectives* 2002; 110(Suppl 4): 565–68.

Repetto, Robert, SB. *Pesticides and the Immune System: The Public Health Risks.* Washington, D.C.: The World Resources Institute, 1996.

Seaton, A. and K. Brown. Increase in Asthma: A More Toxic Environment or a More Susceptible Population? *Thorax* 1994; 49(2): 171–74.

Sly, R. Changing Prevalence of Allergic Rhinitis and Asthma. *Annals of Allergy, Asthma & Immunology* 1999; 82(3): 248–52.

Thickett, K. M. et al. Occupational Asthma Caused by Chloramines in Indoor Swimming-pool Air. *Journal of Alternative and Complementary Medicine* 2002; 19(5): 827–32.

World Health Organization (WHO). Bronchial Asthma. WHO Fact Sheet No. 206, 2000.

CHAPTER 6. Neurological Disorders

Anger, W. Neurobehavioural Testing of Chemicals: Impact in Recommended Standards. *Neurobehavioral Toxicology and Teratology* 1984; 6(2): 147–53.

Baker, E. L. et al. Occupational Lead Neurotoxicity: A Behavioural and Electrophysiological Evaluation. Study Design and Year One Results. *British Journal of Industrial Medicine* 1984; 41(3): 352–61.

————. The Role of Occupational Lead Exposure in the Genesis of Psychiatric and Behavioral Disturbances. *Acta Psychiatrica Scandinavica Supplementum* 1983; 303: 38–48.

Baldi, I. et al. Neuropsychologic Effects of Long-term Exposure to Pesticides: Results from the French Phytoner Study. *Environmental Health Perspectives* 2001; 109(8): 839–44.

Gottwald, B. et al. "Amalgam Disease"—Poisoning, Allergy, or Psychic Disorder? *International Journal of Hygiene and Environmental Health* 2001; 204(4): 223–29.

Gout, O. Vaccinations and Multiple Sclerosis. *Neurological Sciences* 2001; 22(2): 151–54.

Ingalls, T. Endemic Clustering of Multiple Sclerosis in Galion, Ohio, 1982–1985. *The American Journal of Forensic Medicine and Pathology* 1989; 10(3): 213–15.

————. Endemic Clustering of Multiple Sclerosis in Time and Place, 1934–1984. Confirmation of a Hypothesis. *The American Journal of Forensic Medicine and Pathology* 1986; 7(1): 3–8.

Kaplan, B. J. et al. Effective Mood Stabilization with a Chelated Mineral Supplement: An Open-label Trial in Bipolar Disorder. *The Journal of Clinical Psychiatry* 2001; 62(12): 936–44.

Kukull, W. A. Dementia Epidemiology. *The Medical Clinics of North America* 2002; 86(3): 573–90.

Lindh, U. et al. Removal of Dental Amalgam and Other Metal Alloys Supported by Antioxidant Therapy Alleviates Symptoms and Improves Quality of Life in Patients with Amalgam-associated Ill Health. *Neuroendocrinology Letters* 2002; 23(5–6): 459–82.

Morrow, L. A. et al. Neuropsychological Assessment, Depression, and Past Exposure to Organic Solvents. *Applied Neuropsychology* 2001; 8(2): 65–73.

Nishiwaki, Y. et al. Effects of Sarin on the Nervous System in Rescue Team Staff Members and Police Officers 3 Years after the Tokyo Subway Sarin Attack. *Environmental Health Perspectives* 2001; 109(11): 1169–73.

Rea W. Chemical Sensitivities 1995; 3: 1772–75.

Rehner, T. A. et al. Depression among Victims of South Mississippi's Methyl Parathion Disaster. *Health & Social Work* 2000; 25(1): 33–40.

Riise, T., and K. R. Kyvik. Organic Solvents and the Risk of Multiple Sclerosis. *Epidemiology* 2002; 13(6): 718–20.

Schoenthaler, S. J. et al. The Effect of Vitamin-Mineral Supplementation on the Intelligence of American Schoolchildren: A Randomized, Double-blind Placebo-controlled Trial. *Journal of Alternative and Complementary Medicine* 2000; 6(1): 19–29.

———. The Effect of Vitamin-Mineral Supplementation on Juvenile Delinquency among American Schoolchildren: A Randomized, Double-blind Placebo-controlled Trial. *Journal of Alternative and Complementary Medicine* 2000; 6(1): 7–17.

Siblerud, R. A Comparison of Mental Health of Multiple Sclerosis Patients with Silver/Mercury Dental Fillings and Those with Fillings Removed. *Psychological Reports* 1992; 70 (3 Pt 2): 1139–51.

Smialek, P. J. The Investigation of Alleged Insecticide Toxicity: A Case Involving Chlordane Exposure, Multiple Sclerosis, and Peripheral Neuropathy. *Journal of Forensic Sciences* 1986; 31(4): 1499–504.

Snyder, J. W. et al. Acute Manic Psychosis following the Dermal Application of N,N-diethyl-m-toluamide (DEET) in an Adult. *Journal of Toxicology, Clinical Toxicology* 1986; 24(5): 429–39.

Thiruchelvam, M. et al. Developmental Exposure to the Pesticides Paraquat and Maneb and the Parkinson's Disease Phenotype. *Neurotoxicology* 2002; 23(4–5): 621–33.

Whitlock, F. A. Drugs and Depression. *Drugs* 1978; 15(1): 53–71.

Wynn, V. Vitamins and Oral Contraceptive Use. *Lancet* 1975; 1(7906): 561–64.

CHAPTER 7. Digestive Disorders

Armitage, E. et al. Increasing Incidence of Both Juvenile-onset Crohn's Disease and Ulcerative Colitis in Scotland. *European Journal of Gastroenterology & Hepatology* 2001; 13(12): 1439–47.

Colombel, J. F. [Etiology of Crohn's Disease. Current Data.] *La Presse medicale* 1994; 23(12): 558–60.

Crohn's Disease. *The Proceedings of the Nutrition Society* 2002; 61(1): 123–30.

Guo, X. et al. Involvement of Neutrophils and Free Radicals in the Potentiating Effects of Passive Cigarette Smoking on Inflammatory Bowel Disease in Rats. *Gastroenterology* 1999; 117(4): 884–92.

Hijazi, N., and A. Seaton. Diet and Childhood Asthma in a Society in Transition: A Study in Urban and Rural Saudi Arabia. *Thorax* 2000; 55(9); 775–79.

Krzystyniak, K., and M. Fournier. Approaches to the Evaluation of Chemical-induced Immunotoxicity. *Environmental Health Perspectives* 1995; 103(Suppl 9): 17–22.

Lomer, M. C., and J. J. Powell. Fine and Ultrafine Particles of the Diet: Influence on the Mucosal Immune Response and Association with Crohn's Disease. The Proceedings of the Nutrition Society 2002 Feb; 61(1): 123–30.

Mahmud, N. The Urban Diet and Crohn's Disease: Is There a Relationship? *European Journal of Gastroenterology & Hepatology* 2001; 13(2): 93–95.

Miller, C. The Compelling Anomaly of Chemical Intolerance. *Annals of the New York Academy of Sciences* 2001; 933: 1–23.

Smith, C. J., and D. J. Doolittle. An International Literature Survey of "IARC Group I Carcinogens" Reported in Mainstream Cigarette Smoke. *Food and Chemical Toxicology* 1997; 35(10–11): 1107–30.

CHAPTER 8. Hormonal Imbalances

Alleva, E. A. Statement from the Work Session on Environmental Endocrine-disrupting Chemicals: Neural, Endocrine, and Behavioural Effects. *Toxicology and Industrial Health* 1998; 14(1–2): 1–7.

Bener, A. et al. Association between Blood Levels of Lead, Blood Pressure, and Risk of Diabetes and Heart Disease in Workers. *International Archives of Occupational and Environmental Health* 2001; 74(5): 375–78.

Choy, C. M. et al. Infertility, Blood Mercury Concentrations and Dietary Seafood Consumption: A Case-control Study. *BJOG: An*

International Journal of Obstetrics and Gynaecology 2002; 109(10): 1121–25.

Fahey, T. I., and L. Delbridge. Increasing Incidence and Changing Presentation of Thyroid Cancer over a 30-year Period. *The British Journal of Surgery* 1995; 82(4): 518–20.

Gaitan, E. Endemic Goiter in Western Colombia. *Ecology of Disease* 1983; 2(4): 295–308.

Ghinea, E., and M. Oprescu. Studies on the Action of Pesticides upon the Endocrines Using In Vitro Human Thyroid Cells Culture and In Vivo Animal Models. I. Herbicides—Aminotriasole (amitrol) and Atrazine. *Endocrinologie* 1979; 17(3): 185–90.

Gist, G. L. Benzene—A Review of the Literature from a Health Effects Perspective. *Toxicology and Industrial Health* 1997; 13(6):661–714.

Glynn, A. W. et al. Organochlorines in Swedish Women: Determinants of Serum Concentrations. *Environmental Health Perspectives* 2003; 111(3): 349–55.

Heeremans, A. et al. Elimination Profile of Methylthiouracil in Cows after Oral Administration. *Analyst* 1988; 123(12): 2629–32.

Ho, E. et al. Dietary Zinc Supplementation Inhibits NFkappaB Activation and Protects against Chemically Induced Diabetes in CD1 Mice. *Experimental Biology and Medicine* (*Maywood*) 2001; 226(2): 103–11.

Kosuda, L. L., and P. E. Bigazzi. Effects of HgC12 on the Expression of Autoimmune Responses and Disease in Diabetes-prone (DP) BB Rats. *Autoimmunity* 1997; 26(3): 173–87.

Krivosheeva, S. S. et al. [Effects of Working Conditions in the Production of Synthetic Rubber on Workers' Health.] *Gigiena i Sanitariia* 2001; 3: 47–49.

Lissner, L. et al. Body Weight Variability in Men: Metabolic Rate, Health, and Longevity. *International Journal of Obesity* 1990; 14(4): 373–83.

Mesaros-Kanjski, E. et al. Endemic Goiter and Plasmatic Levels of Vitamins A and E in the Schoolchildren on the Island of Kirk, Croatia. *Collegium Antropologicum* 1999; 23(2): 729–36.

Muir, T. Societal Costs of Exposure to Toxic Substances: Economic and Health Costs of Four Case Studies That Are Candidates for

Environmental Causation. *Health Perspectives* 2001; 109(Suppl 6): 885–903.

Sala, M. et al. Association between Serum Concentrations of Hexa-chlorobenzene and Polychlorobiphenyls with Thyroid Hormone and Liver Enzymes in a Sample of the General Population. *Occupational and Environmental Medicine* 2001; 58(3): 172–77.

Shobha, T. R. Glycosuria in Organophosphate and Carbamate Poisoning. *The Journal of the Association of Physicians of India* 2000; 48(12): 1197–99.

Slutsky, M., and B. S. Levy. Azoospermia and Oligospermia among a Large Cohort of DBCP Applicators in 12 Countries. *International Journal of Occupational Medicine and Environmental Health* 1999; 5(2): 116–22.

Tiemann, U. Influence of Organochlorine Pesticides on ATPase Activities of Microsomal Fractions of Bovine Oviductal and Endometrial Cells. *Toxicology Letters* 1999; 104(1–2): 75–81.

Veeramachaneni, D. Deteriorating Trends in Male Reproduction: Idiopathic or Environmental? *Animal Reproduction Science* 2000; 60–61: 121–130.

Vena, J. et al. Exposure to Dioxin and Nonneoplastic Mortality in the Expanded IARC International Cohort Study of Phenoxy Herbicide and Chlorophenol Production Workers and Sprayers. *Environmental Health Perspectives* 1998; 106(Suppl 2): 645–53.

Wong, G. W. Increasing Incidence of Childhood Grave's Disease in Hong Kong: A Follow-up Study. *Clinical Endocrinology* 2001; 54(4): 547–50.

Younglai, E. V. et al. Levels of Environmental Contaminants in Human Follicular Fluid, Serum, and Seminal Plasma of Couples Undergoing In Vitro Fertilization. *Archives of Environmental Contamination and Toxicology* 2002; 43(1): 121–26.

CHAPTER 9. Cardiovascular Diseases

Bener, A. et al. Association between Blood Levels of Lead, Blood Pressure, and Risk of Diabetes and Heart Disease in Workers. *International*

Archives of Occupational and Environmental Health 2001; 74(5): 375–78.

Carvalho, W. Risk Factors Related with Occupational and Environmental Exposure to Organochlorine Insecticides in the State of Bahia, Brazil, 1985. *Boletin de la Oficina Sanitaria Panamericana* 1991; 111(6): 512–24.

Cedergren, M. I. et al. Chlorination By-products and Nitrate in Drinking Water and Risk for Congenital Cardiac Defects. *Environmental Research* 2002; 89(2): 124–30.

Guloglu, C., and P. G. Erten. Acute Accidental Exposure to Chlorine Gas in the Southeast of Turkey: A Study of 106 Cases. *Environmental Research* 2002; 88(2): 89–93.

Hill, W. D. et al. The NF-kappaB Inhibitor Diethyldithiocarbamate (DDTC) Increases Brain Cell Death in a Transient Middle Cerebral Artery Occlusion Model of Ischemia. *Brain Research Bulletin* 2001; 55(3): 375–86.

Hollis, G. Organophosphate Poisoning versus Brainstem Stroke. *The Medical Journal of Australia* 1999; 170(12): 596–97.

Hong, Y. C. et al. Air Pollution: A New Risk Factor in Ischemic Stroke Mortality. *Stroke* 2002; 33(9): 2165–69.

Hooiveld, M. et al. Second Follow-up of a Dutch Cohort Occupationally Exposed to Phenoxy Herbicides, Chlorophenols, and Contaminants. *American Journal of Epidemiology* 1998; 147(9): 891–901.

Kinoshita, H. et al. [A Case of Carbamate Poisoning in which GCMS Was Useful to Identify Causal Substance and to Decide the Appropriate Treatment.] *Chudoku Kenkyukai Jun Kikanshi* 2001; 14(4): 343–46.

Klatsky, A. L. Alcohol and Cardiovascular Diseases: A Historical Overview. *Annals of the New York Academy of Sciences* 2002; 957: 7–15.

Kundiev, Y. I. Actual Medical and Ergonomic Problems in Agriculture in the Ukraine. *International Journal of Occupational Medicine and Environmental Health* 1994; 7(1): 3–11.

Kurth, T. et al. Smoking and the Risk of Hemorrhagic Stroke in Men. *Stroke* 2003; 34(5): 1151–55.

Laden, F. et al. Predictors of Plasma Concentrations of DDE and PCBs in a Group of U.S. Women. *Environmental Health Perspectives* 1999; 107(1): 75–81.

Laplanche, A. et al. Exposure to Vinyl Chloride Monomer: Results of a Cohort Study after a Seven Year Follow-Up. The French VCM Group. *British Journal of Industrial Medicine* 1992; 49(2): 134–37.

Marek, K. et al. Examination of Health Effects after Exposure to Metallic Mercury Vapors in Workers Engaged in Production of Chlorine and Acetic Aldehyde. I. Evaluation of General Health Status. *Heavy metals* 1995; 46(2): 101–109.

Maschewsky, W. [Do Workplace Chemicals Harm the Heart?] *Sozial-Und Praventivmedizin* 1993; 38(2): 71–76.

Meltzer, H. M. et al. Does Dietary Arsenic and Mercury Affect Cutaneous Bleeding Time and Blood Lipids in Humans? *Biological Trace Element Research* 1994; 46(1–2): 135–53.

Morgan, D. P., and H. H. Saikaly. Morbidity and Mortality in Workers Occupationally Exposed to Pesticides. *Archives of Environmental Contamination and Toxicology* 1980; 9(3): 349–82.

Mukamal, K. Alcohol Use and Prognosis in Patients with Coronary Heart Disease. *Preventive Cardiology* 2003; 6(2): 93–98.

Nikiforov, B. et al. [Heavy Metal Exposure of the Population in an Area of Nonferrous Metallurgy—A Prerequisite for the Development of Atherosclerotic Diseases] *Problemi Na Khigienata* 1987; 12: 27–37.

Saadeh, A. M. et al. Cardiac Manifestations of Acute Carbamate and Organophosphate Poisoning. *Heart* 1997; 77(5): 461–64.

Sauviat, M. P. [Cardiotoxicity of Lindane, a Gamma Isomer of Hexachlorocyclohexane.] *Journal de la Societe de Biologie* 2002; 196(4): 339–48.

Shindell, S. Mortality of Workers Employed in the Manufacture of Chlordane: An Update. *Journal of Occupational Medicine* 1986; 28(7): 497–501.

Taylor, A. E. Cardiovascular Effects of Environmental Chemicals. *Otolaryngology and Head and Neck Surgery* 1996; 114(2): 209–11.

Tollestrup, K., and J. Allard. Mortality in a Cohort of Orchard Workers Exposed to Lead Arsenate Pesticide Spray. *Archives of Environmental Health* 1995; 50(3): 221–29.

Toren, K., and H. Westberg. Health Effects of Working in Pulp and Paper Mills: Exposure, Obstructive Airways Diseases, Hypersensitivity Reactions, and Cardiovascular Diseases. *American Journal of Industrial Medicine* 1996; 29(2): 111–22.

Walsh, L. P., and D. M. Stocco. Dimethoate Inhibits Steroidogenesis by Disrupting Transcription of the Steroidogenic Acute Regulatory Development of Atherosclerotic Diseases. *Problemi Na Khigienata* 1987; 12: 27–37.

Wang, C. H. et al. Biological Gradient between Long-term Arsenic Exposure and Carotid Atherosclerosis. *Circulation* 2002; 105(15): 1804–89.

Weihe, P. et al. [Environmental Epidemiology Research Leads to a Decrease of the Exposure Limit for Mercury.] *Ugeskrift for Laeger* 2003; 165(2): 107–11.

Zeighami, E. A., and G. F. Craun. Chlorination, Water Hardness and Serum Cholesterol in Forty-six Wisconsin Communities. *International Journal of Epidemiology* 1990; 19(1): 49–58.

CHAPTER 10. Cancer

Baris, D. Epidemiology of Lymphomas. *Current Opinion in Oncology* 2000; 12(5): 383–94.

Connecticut State Employees Association. *Please Allow Me to Introduce Myself: Cancer-Causing Chemicals in the Workplace.* Occupational Safety and Health Department, 143 Washington Avenue, Albany, NY 12210. (This document is found at www.csea801.org/cancerchems.pdf.)

Costantini, A. S. et al. A Multicenter Case-control Study in Italy on Hematolymphopoietic Neoplasms and Occupation. *Epidemiology* 2001; 12(1): 78–87.

Dodds, E. L. Synthetic Oestrogenic Agents without the Phenanthrene Nucleus. *Nature* 1936.

Gottlieb, M. S. Case-control Cancer Mortality Study and Chlorination of Drinking Water in Louisiana. *Environmental Health Perspectives* 1982; 46: 169–77.

Korach, K. S. et al. Xenoestrogens and Estrogen Receptor Action. In John Thomas, ed. *Endocrine Toxicology,* 2nd ed. Washington, DC: Taylor and Francis, 1997.

Wetherill, Y. B. et al. The Xenoestrogen Bisphenol A Induces Inappropriate Androgen Receptor Activation and Mitogenesis in Prostatic Adenocarcinoma Cells. *Molecular Cancer Therapeutics* 2002; 1(7): 515–24.

CHAPTER 11. Multiple Chemical Sensitivity

Black, D. W. et al. Multiple Chemical Sensitivity Syndrome: Symptom Prevalence and Risk Factors in a Military Population. *Archives of Internal Medicine* 2000; 160(8): 1169–76.

Kreutzer, R., and N. Lashuay. Prevalence of People Reporting Sensitivities to Chemicals in a Population-based Survey. *American Journal of Epidemiology* 1999; 150(1): 1–12.

Miller, C. S. Chemical Sensitivity Attributed to Pesticide Exposure versus Remodeling. *Archives of Environmental Health* 1995; 50(2): 119–29.

Schumm, W. R. et al. Self-reported Changes in Subjective Health and Anthrax Vaccination as Reported by Over 900 Persian Gulf War Era Veterans. *Psychological Reports* 2002; 90(2): 639–53.

CHAPTER 12. Obesity and Muskuloskeletal Disorders

Baillie-Hamilton, P. Chemical Toxins: A Hypothesis to Explain the Global Obesity Epidemic. *Journal of Alternative and Complementary Medicine* 2002; 8(2): 185–92.

Bell, I. R., and G. E. Schwartz. Illness from Low Levels of Environmental Chemicals: Relevance to Chronic Fatigue Syndrome and Fibromyalgia. *The American Journal of Medicine* 1998; 105(3A): 74S–82S.

Bjorntorp P. Endocrine Abnormalities of Obesity. *Metabolism* 1995; 44(9 Suppl): 21–23.

Evengard, B. Chronic Fatigue Syndrome: Probable Pathogenesis and Possible Treatments. *Drugs* 2002; 62(17): 2433–46.

Galland, L. Magnesium and Immune Function: An Overview. *Magnesium* 1988; 7(5–6): 290–99.

Lohmann, K., and E. Schwarz. [Multiple Chemical Sensitivity Disorder in Patients with Neurotoxic Illnesses.] *Gesundheitswesen* 1996; 58(6): 322–16.

Mayes, M. Epidemiologic Studies of Environmental Agents and Systemic Autoimmune Diseases. *Environmental Health Perspectives* 1999; 107(Suppl 5): 743–48.

McCauley, L. A. et al. Chronic Fatigue in a Population-based Study of Gulf War Veterans. *Archives of Environmental Health* 2002; 57(4): 340–48.

Pedersen, L. M. Rheumatic Disease, Heavy-metal Pigments, and the Great Masters. *Lancet* 1988; 1(8597): 1267–69.

Tahmaz, N., and J. W. Cherrie. Chronic Fatigue and Organophosphate Pesticides in Sheep Farming: A Retrospective Study Amongst People Reporting to a UK Pharmacovigilance Scheme. *The Annals of Occupational Hygiene* 2003; 47(4): 261–67.

Tapiero, H., and K. D. Tew. Estrogens and Environmental Estrogens. *Biomedicine & Pharmacotherapy* 2002; 56(1): 36–44.

Thompson, A. E., and J. E. Pope. Increased Prevalence of Scleroderma in Southwestern Ontario: A Cluster Analysis. *The Journal of Rheumatology* 2002; 29(9): 1867–73.

Villeneuve, D. C. et al. Effect of Food Deprivation on Low-Level Hexachlorobenzene Exposure in Rats. *The Science of the Total Environment* 1977; 8(2): 179–86.

CHAPTER 13. Childhood Disorders

Capel, I.D. et al. Comparison of Concentrations of Some Trace, Bulk, and Toxic Metals in the Hair of Normal and Dyslexic Children. *Clinical Chemistry* 1981; 27(6): 879–81.

Collins, V. Scots Study on Autism Poses New Question of MMR Link. *The Herald* (Glasgow) 22 July 2002.

Geier, D. A. A Comparative Evaluation of the Effects of MMR Immunization and Mercury Doses from Thimerosal-Containing Childhood Vaccines on the Population Prevalence of Autism. *Medical Science Monitor* 2004; 10(3): 133–39.

Glotzer, D. E., and H. Bauchner. Management of Childhood Lead Poisoning: Clinical Impact and Cost-effectiveness: *Medical Decision Making* 1995; 15(1): 13–24.

He, Y., and F. Xu. [Application of Conners Rating Scales in the Study of Lead Exposure and Behavioral Effects in Children.] *Zhonghua Yu Fang Yi Xue Za Zhi* 2003; 34(5): 290–93.

Ingram, J. L. et al. Prenatal Exposure of Rats to Valproic Acid Reproduces the Cerebellar Anomalies Associated with Autism. *Neurotoxicol Teratol* 2000; 22(3): 319–24.

Kidd, P. Attention Deficit/Hyperactivity Disorder (ADHD) in Children: Rationale for Its Integrative Management. *Alternative Medicine Review: A Journal of Clinical Therapeutic* 2000; 5(5): 402–28.

Leonard, C. M. et al. Anatomical Risk Factors that Distinguish Dyslexia from SLI Predict Reading Skill in Normal Children. *Journal of Communication Disorders* 2002; 35(6): 501–31.

Rice, D. Critical Periods of Vulnerability for the Developing Nervous System: Evidence from Humans and Animal Models. *Environmental Health Perspectives* 2000; 108(Suppl 3): 511–33.

Sowell, E. R. et al. Cortical Abnormalities in Children and Adolescents with Attention-Deficit Hyperactivity Disorder. *Lancet* 2003; 362(9397): 1699–707.

Stein, J. et al. In Harm's Way: Toxic Threats to Child Development. *Journal of Developmental and Behavioral Pediatrics* 2002; 23(1 Suppl): S13–22.

Weihe, P. et al. [Environmental Epidemiology Research Leads to a Decrease of the Exposure Limit for Mercury.] *Ugeskrift for Laeger* 2003; 165(2): 107–11.

Index

About the Author

DR. PAULA BAILLIE-HAMILTON is a medical doctor and has previously worked in the following fields: cardiology, gastroenterology, rheumatology, pediatrics, emergency medicine, psychiatry, obstetrics and gynecology, endocrinology, oncology, general medicine, and general surgery. She also holds an academic doctorate for her research into the effects of toxic chemicals on human health at Christ Church, Oxford University.

She is now a Visiting Fellow in Occupational and Environmental Health at Stirling University in Scotland. She is also a full member of the British Society for Allergy, Environmental, and Nutritional Medicine. One of England's foremost experts on toxic chemicals and their harmful effects on our health, she has published full papers in international academic journals in this field.

Her first book, *The Body Restoration Plan* (Penguin, 2003), was first published in the UK in 2002 as *The Detox Diet*. The book has also been translated into Dutch and German and, to date, over 250,000 copies are in print. She now is the health correspondent for the U.S.-based magazine *Phenomena*.